Oncogenes in Cancer Diagnosis

Contributions to Oncology
Beiträge zur Onkologie

Vol. 39

Series Editors
J. H. Holzner, Wien; *W. Queißer,* Mannheim

KARGER

Basel · München · Paris · London · New York · New Dehli · Bangkok · Singapore · Tokyo · Sydney

Oncogenes in Cancer Diagnosis

Volume Editors
C.R. Bartram, Ulm; *K. Munk,* Heidelberg; *M. Schwab,* Heidelberg

36 figures and 11 tables, 1990

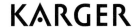

KARGER

Basel · München · Paris · London · New York · New Dehli · Bangkok · Singapore · Tokyo · Sydney

Contributions to Oncology
Beiträge zur Onkologie

Drug Dosage
The authors and the publisher have exerted every effort to ensure that drug selection and dosage set forth in this text are in accord with current recommendations and practice at the time of publication. However, in view of ongoing research, changes in government regulations, and the constant flow of information relating to drug therapy and drug reactions, the reader is urged to check the package insert for each drug for any change in indications and dosage and for added warnings and precautions. This is particularly important when the recommended agent is a new and/or infrequently employed drug.

© Copyright 1990 by S. Karger GmbH, P.O. Box 1724, D-8034 Germering/München and S. Karger AG, Postfach, CH-4009 Basel
Printed in Germany by Bonitas-Bauer, Würzburg
ISBN 3-8055-5231-9

Contents

Recessive Genetic Alterations

Diagnostic Aspects

Preface

The topic of the VII. INTERNATIONAL EXPERT MEETING of the *Dr. Mildred Scheel Stiftung für Krebsforschung* was 'Oncogenes and Their Significance in Tumor Diagnosis'. The Dr. Mildred Scheel Stiftung, founded by Dr. Mildred Scheel in 1976, is organizing expert meetings in two year intervals. The purpose of these meetings is to bring together internationally renowned scientists for discussions of recent progress in cancer research and at the same time to identify the most promising developments that would merit priority funding. The funds that are made available to investigators come exclusively from private donations. It is understandable, therefore, that the donors expect grants to be provided only for the most innovative and promising projects in cancer research. To assure the most efficient allocation of funds the close discussion between experts of the international scientific community, German scientists and both the Scientific Advisory Committee and the Executive Board of the Dr. Mildred Scheel Stiftung is an important instrument. The scientific presentations of the Expert Meeting are compiled and published in the series 'Contributions to Oncology' aiming to inform interested basic scientists and clinicians about topical developments in cancer research.

The VII. Expert Meeting has brought together scientists to discuss the increasingly apparent role that cellular genes have in the genesis of human cancers and to evaluate possibilities for employing the knowledge that has accrued as diagnostic and prognostic parameters. There is evidence now that alterations of cellular genes are instrumental for tumor development. Human cancer appears to be the result of a genetic accident in the cell. The significance of cellular genes in tumorigenesis has been known since long, but their molecular identity has been enigmatic until the experimental tools were available to perform molecular genome analyses. Today approximately 60 cancer-related genes are known that occupy central positions in normal processes of signal transduction, differentiation and development.

Cancer-related cellular genes may acquire oncogenic potential in two principally different ways. First, cellular genes can assume an abnormal function. Mechanisms that have been identified are a) mutations resulting in an altered protein; b) chromosomal translocations leading to aberrant expression or structural changes of the gene; and c) amplification resulting in the selective increase of the number of gene copies. According to prevailing terminology the normal gene is referred to as the proto-oncogene, the abnormal gene as the oncogene. Second, the function of a cellular gene may be lost. The prime mechanisms resulting in loss of gene function appear to be a) mutation causing gene inactivation, and b) deletion from the genome. The intact normal gene obviously is involved in maintaining the normal growth pattern of the cell and for this reason is referred to as tumor-suppressorgene.

Cancer cells usually do not carry a single alteration but rather are characterized by a combination of different types of genetic changes. In spite of this, alterations of a specific gene may serve as molecular hallmarks of a particular type of cancer. For instance, chronic myelogenous leukemia (CML) is signified by a characteristic translocation involving the *ABL* oncogene. This genetic alteration has gained great clinical significance for the diagnosis of CML and the monitoring of the therapeutic effectiviness. And in neuroblastoma and breast cancer the amplification of the oncogenes *MYCN* and *ERBB*2, respectively, is found in particularly aggressively growing forms of cancer. In these cases amplification has turned out to be a genetic parameter of early predictive value of future tumor growth.

Oncogenes and tumor-suppressor genes are two groups of cancer-related genes that have opened the door for an understanding of molecular mechanisms contributing to human cancers. Some members of these groups of genes had their clinical debut and add to the available spectrum of diagnostic and prognostic possibilities. It is to be expected that further promotion of research directed at identifying the role of cancer-related genes will have far-reaching consequences for diagnosis, prognosis and most likely for the therapy of human cancer.

C.R. Bartram
K. Munk
M. Schwab

Contrib Oncol. vol 39, pp 1–9 (Karger, Basel 1990)

A Major Decision: Proliferation or Differentiation. Interactions Between Pathway-specific Transcription Factors Exemplify a Molecular Mechanism for the Decision

P. Herrlich, C. Jonat, H. Ponta, H. J. Rahmsdorf

Kernforschungszentrum Karlsruhe, Institut für Genetik und Toxikologie, and Universität Karlsruhe, Institut für Genetik, Karlsruhe, FRG

During development and throughout life of a multicellular organism, there are always cells that need to go through the decision between continued self-renewal and differentiation. Features of the microenvironment such as cell-cell contact, growth factors and hormones are likely to determine which route a cell will follow. While basic fibroblast growth factor and other growth factors keep adipogenic cells, myoblasts and mammary epithelial stem cells in self-renewal, confluence and specific hormones trigger differentiation [3, 16, 21]. One of these hormones is cortisol. These points of commitment seem vulnerable to cancerogenic transformation. In cancer cells the conditions for self-renewal predominate although reversal of the 'decision' may still be possible by application of so called biological response modifiers such as retinoic acid. Also the precancerous development is influenced by the interplay of conditions favoring either proliferation or differentiation. In experimental mouse skin carcinogenesis, phorbol ester tumor promoters act as potent mitogens inducing the promotion phenotype that represents a state of increased risk towards the generation of papillomas. The cortisol analogue dexamethasone effectively obliterates both the proliferation and the promotion phenotype, and it induces hormone dependent differentiation [2]. Investigations into the mechanism of phorbol ester action and of its block by dexamethasone have revealed the molecular details of one of the decision mechanisms. The transcription factor responsible for part or all of the proliferation and promotion pathway is blocked directly by interaction with the differentiation-specific transcription factor [12]. Interestingly the reverse is true as well: possibly based on the same interaction, the differentiation pathway is reversed by activating the proliferation related program. Conditions of interference with one pathway do not automatically turn on the other pathway. The decision process occurs in several steps.

Indicator Genes

A program that drives cells to self-renewal and tumor promotion must consist of gene products that differ from those needed for differentiation and antipromotion. A switch mechanism as postulated above, is likely to change the program of genes expressed. For a study of the mechanism, indicator genes specific for the two pathways are required. Based on information of previous experiments [1, 10, 15], two indicator genes were chosen: a gene carrying promoter elements of the human collagenase gene representing a genetic structure that responds to phorbol esters and growth factors, and a promoter-gene construct with a glucocorticoid hormone responsive element (GRE) (fig. 1). The collagenase promoter is transcribed upon posttranslational activation of the transcription factor AP-1 [1, 14]. This factor consists of two subunits that are coded for by the cellular oncogenes c-*jun* and c-*fos* (e. g. reviewed in [4]), and it binds to the promoter element TRE (TPA responsive element; 5′TGAGTCA3′). The promoter carrying the GRE sequence 5′GGTACAnnnTGTTCT3′ is induced by interacting with another transcription factor, the glucocorticoid hormone recep-

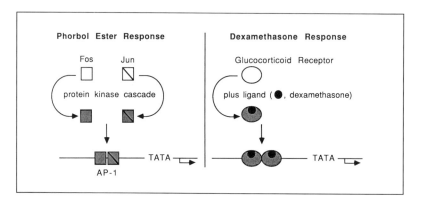

Fig. 1. Transcription factors and cis-acting elements acting in two different pathways: Phorbol esters induce the expression of a number of genes characteristic of proliferating cells. AP-1 is responsible for part of this regulation, but probably not for the preparation of S phase. Dexamethasone induces the hormone dependent differentiation program.

tor [18]. To bind at the GRE, the receptor requires activation by the ligand (e. g. by dexamethasone).

To imitate the switch situation and to study the interference between conditions favoring the 'proliferation program' and others that induce differentiation, we examine the phorbol ester response of the collagenase promoter in the presence of dexamethasone, and, conversely, the hormone response of the GRE-driven promoter under conditions indicative of proliferation. For reasons that will become clear, this latter condition is generated by establishing elevated levels of the activated transcription factor AP-1 (Fos/Jun).

The TRE Confers Responsiveness Both to Phorbol Ester Dependent Transcription and to Dexamethasone Dependent Downregulation

Phorbol esters cause a massive change of cellular behavior and morphology. The multicellular inflammatory response of mouse skin to phorbol ester treatment is extinguished by the presence of dexamethasone. In mouse epidermis as well as in various cultured cells, phorbol esters induce the expression of a large number of genes many of which are characteristic of proliferating cells [6]. The promoter element TRE has been one of the first discovered as phorbol ester responsive. It binds the heterodimeric complex Fos/Jun. Fos/Jun indeed participates in the proliferative response of cells since it represents a target transcription factor for growth factor and oncogene induced signal transduction pathways [8]. The collagenase promoter is largely regulated through its TRE, and AP-1 (Fos/Jun) is the limiting component in the transcriptional activation [12]. AP-1 is responsible for both the basal and the phorbol ester induced transcription.

The collagenase promoter is not only activated by phorbol esters but also downregulated by dexamethasone. Thus its regulation behaves as is expected for an effector gene controlled by a switch mechanism. The correlation between promoter regulation and the cellular phenotype makes the mechanism a prime candidate for the decision between tumor promotion and antipromotion: AP-1 activity representing the determinant of tumor promotion. Both activation and the inhibition by dexamethasone occur in the presence or absence of inhibitors of protein synthesis indicating that the regulation depends only on preexisting components. A thorough mutational analysis of the collagenase promoter and the study of various promoter constructs has now shown that both phorbol ester induced promoter activation and dexamethasone-dependent inhibition of transcription require the presence of the TRE sequence and nothing but the TRE within a minimal promoter [12]. Thus the TRE and the transcription factor AP-1 must be targets of the phorbol ester induced activation and of the downregulation by dexamethasone.

A Novel Type of Action of the Hormone Receptor

In receptor deficient CV-1 cells, the indicator gene driven by the collagenase promoter can be induced by phorbol ester but cannot be repressed by hormone. Repression is reestablished upon expressing the receptor through transfecting a suitable cDNA clone. Thus the hormone receptor protein is required for the negative action just as for the positive one. This experimental set-up permits to assay various receptor mutants for their ability to repress the collagenase promoter, and has revealed that the receptor protein does not need to bind to DNA for its repressing function. This represents a yet unrecognized action of the hormone receptor. While the activation of genes by the hormone receptor requires binding of the receptor to the GRE element and contact between the receptor's transactivating domain with the transcriptional initiation complex, repression is exerted without direct binding to DNA.

The novel type of action is underlined by a completely different hormone dose dependence. About 20 fold less hormone induces half-maximal repression than is required for half-maximal induction of the GRE containing promoter. Repression is in fact established at hormone concentrations within the range of the daily fluctuations in the human organism. Repression does, therefore, not automatically involve the induction of the hormone dependent genetic program which is an interesting facet of the molecular switch mechanism (see fig. 2). The GRE-linked promoters are induced at much higher levels of hormone: those that are reached under stress conditions.

Interestingly we found genes that both carry GREs and are phorbol ester inducible and hormone repressible. Thus the transcriptional activity of these genes is a function of the net effect of positive and negative actions on the same promoter. Over the physiological range of hormone levels, the proliferation-related function of these genes is modulated, while at stress levels the genes are induced through the dominating GRE element. Genes with such dual control include c-*jun* and metallothionein IIA. The GRE element in c-*jun* has as yet not been localized.

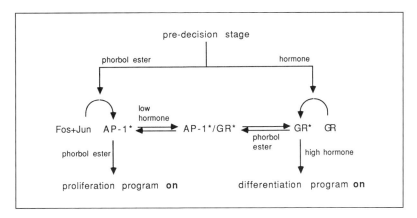

Fig. 2. Interference between pathways: a patative mechanism. The decision for a pathway occurs in several steps. In a reversible phase, the decision depends on the relative concentrations of the activated transcription factors AP-1* and GR* (= glucocorticoid receptor). Their interaction is mutually inhibitory. Wether the interaction is direct or involves a third partner is not known. The interaction between the transcription factors may in fact take place at the DNA target, with one factor bound to its cis-acting element (see fig. 1). Subsequent steps may enforce increasing irreversibility, e. g. by getting cells into proliferation (which requires functions in addition to AP-1).

Mechanism of the negative action of dexamethasone

Since the negative regulation by dexamethasone operates with pre-existing protein factors the induction of synthesis of a repressor can be ruled out. The dexamethasone receptor could inactivate AP-1 function by either

- dislodging AP-1 from its site of action (TRE) or
- modifying AP-1 by an as yet unknown enzyme activity or
- inhibiting the transactivating function of AP-1 by stoichiometric interaction.

Dislodging is made unlikely by the low hormone dependence and the fact that the receptor does not need to bind to DNA. Also, promoters carrying the TRE in various neighborhoods, are repressible. No other consensus sequence but the TRE itself is the target. Band-shift experiments with extracts from cells treated with phorbol esters or with phorbol esters plus dexamethasone reveal no difference, that is no extra DNA-protein complex is detected. Only the AP-1/TRE complex is formed. Instead of reducing the binding of AP-1, dexamethasone causes even elevated abundance of AP-1

DNA binding activity. This is due to increased synthesis of both Fos and Jun observed under conditions of simultaneous treatment with phorbol esters and dexamethasone [12].

A careful search for altered modification patterns by dexamethasone of both Fos and Jun has been unsuccessful. Fos and Jun occur in various forms, as judged by migration in denaturing one- and two-dimensional polyacrylamide gels (collaboration with Dr. Marc Timmers, Leiden). Dexamethasone does not alter these patterns. Thus, there is as yet no evidence for a modification of Fos or Jun by the hormone receptor. Rather a stoichiometric protein-protein interaction is probably the molecular basis of the functional inactivation. Complexes of AP-1 with the hormone receptor have been found by direct immune precipitation, by immune precipitation of AP-1 complexes cross-linked to the TRE, and by affinity chromatography on TRE columns. AP-1 is eluted from affinity columns by raising the ion concentration from 0.1 to 0.6 M NaCl. The eluted material contains Jun protein detected by Western blot analysis. Dexamethasone receptor is coeluted if the cells had been pretreated with the hormone but not with extracts from non-treated cells or from cells treated with the hormone analogue RU 486. RU 486 causes nuclear translocation of the receptor and binding of the receptor to GRE elements while blocking both the transactivating and repressing abilities of the hormone receptor.

The molecular association of receptor and AP-1 represents a plausible mechanism of AP-1 downmodulation. Since the association involves two transcription factors both of which are programmed for specific cis-acting elements, we explored whether the association also inactivated the hormone receptor when acting as a positive transcription factor.

Fos and Jun inhibit the positive gene regulatory function of hormone receptor

We now look at the differentiation pathway using the GRE-promoter as the indicator gene. Can differentiation-specific gene expression be reversed by elevated signalling that is typical of proliferating cells? By overexpressing Fos or Jun, the hormone dependent response of a GRE-promoter was severely inhibited (Jonat et al., submitted).Although not proven, the idea is tempting that the complex receptor/AP-1 was inactive in both pathways, with AP-1 as the DNA binding transcription factor, or with the receptor as the 'active' factor. Whether the receptor inactivation is due to protein-

protein interaction or (and) receptor phosphorylation [9] cannot be decided at this time. Clearly, the hormone-induced genetic program can be reversed. In earlier experiments with GRE-oncogene constructs we and others had observed a transient induction by hormone [11, 19]. The transient nature may be caused by the oncogene-driven inactivation of the hormone receptor. Interestingly, reduced binding to cytosolic hepatic hormone receptor of radiolabeled dexamethasone has been found in methylcholanthrene or phenobarbital treated rats [20]. Similarly, tumor promoter in mouse skin appear to reduce receptor levels [5]. These effects are, however, too slow to account for the inhibition of GRE promoter activity observed here.

The implications of the switch mechanism

The suggested mechanism not only permits a stepwise decision process, but also fine regulation depending on the relative levels of the active transcription factors (fig. 2). These relative levels are decisive for the genetic program and may be quite different in different cells. In cells supplied with both phorbol esters and a receptor-saturating dose of dexamethasone, one or the other influence may dominate. For instance in NIH3T3 cells the phorbol ester response prevails [19], while in the mouse skin the hormone enforces antipromotion. Since phorbol ester and dexamethasone act at the same molecular step in transcription, involvement of this step in the development of the promotion phenotype and of its reversal respectively, is made highly probable. The switch mechanism described here may operate at the branching points of various differentiation pathways. In adipocyte differentiation the transcription of a glucocorticoid responsive regulatory gene is suppressed by phorbol esters or basic fibroblast growth factor [16]. Mice that overexpress as a transgene one of a variety of signalling components of the 'proliferation pathway' (e. g. c-myc, c-ras, c-fos) are disturbed in the normal differentiation [7]. Which cell lineage is affected, depends on the transgene and on the promoter. Differentiation systems that have been studied so far, show the stepwise decision mechanism which we have described here. For instance, the turn-off of muscle specific gene expression by basic fibroblast growth factor does not require entry into proliferation [13]. Also in the adipocyte system phorbol esters repress the hormone induced differentiation without causing proliferation [16]. Conversely, muscle-specific gene expression is transiently inducible in the presence of continued cell cycling [17].

We favor the idea that the mitogen-hormone antagony exemplifies the type of molecular switches to be expected but does not represent the only switch mechanism. Rather a combination of several switch mechanisms may be needed for the decision between self-renewal and differentiation.

References

1   Angel P, Baumann I, Stein B, Delius H, Rahmsdorf HJ, Herrlich P: 12-0-tetradeca-noyl-phorbol-13-acetate induction of the human collagenase gene is mediated by an inducible enhancer element located in the 5′-flanking region. Mol Cell Biol 1987; 7:2256–2266.

2   Belman S, Troll W: The inhibition of croton oil-promoted mouse skin tumorigenesis by steroid hormones. Cancer Res 1972;32:450–454.

3   Clegg CH, Linkhart TA, Olwin BB, Hauschka SD: Growth factor control of skeletal muscle differentiation: commitment to terminal differentiation occurs in G1 phase and its repressed by fibroblast growth factor. J Cell Biol 1987;105:949–956.

4   Curran T, Franza Jr BR: Fos and Jun: The AP-1 connection. Cell 1988;55:395–397.

5   Davidson KA, Slaga TJ: Glucocorticoid receptor levels in mouse skin after repetitive applications of 12-O-tetradecanoylphorbol-13-acetate. Cancer Res 1983;43:3847–3851.

6   Denhardt DT, Craig AM, Smith JH: Regulation of gene expression by the tumor promoter 12-O-tetradecanoylphorbol-13-acetate, in Colburn NH (ed): Genes and signal transduction in multistage carcinogenesis, New York, Dekker, 1989, pp 167–189.

7   Hanahan D: Dissecting multistep tumorigenesis in transgenic mice. Ann Rev Genet 1988;22:479–519.

8   Herrlich P, Ponta H: 'Nuclear' oncogenes convert extracellular stimuli into changes in the genetic program. TIG 1989;5:112–116.

9   Hoeck W, Rusconi S, Groner B: Down-regulation and phosphorylation of glucocorticoid receptors in cultured cells. J Biol Chem 1989;264:14396–14402.

10 Hynes N, van Ooyen AJJ, Kennedy N, Herrlich P, Ponta H, Groner B: Subfragments of the large terminal repeat cause glucocorticoid-responsive expression of mouse mammary tumor virus and of an adjacent gene. Proc Natl Acad Sci USA 1983; 80:3637–3641.

11 Jaggi R, Salmons B, Muellener D, Groner B: The v-mos and H-ras oncogene expression represses glucocorticoid hormone-dependent transcription from the mouse mammary tumor virus LTR. EMBO J 1986;5:2609–2616.

12 Jonat C, Stein B, Ponta H, Herrlich P, Rahmsdorf HJ: Positive and negative regulation of collagenase expression, in Birkedal-Hansen H, Werb 7, Welgus H, van Wart H (eds): Matrix Metalloproteinases and Inhibitors. Stuttgart, Fischer, 1190.

13 Lathrop B, Olson E, Glaser L: Control by fibroblast growth factor of differentiation in the BC3H1 muscle cell line. J Cell Biol 1985;100:1540–1547.

14 Lee W, Mitchell P, Tjian R: Purified transcription factor AP-1 interacts with TPA-inducible enhancer elements. Cell 1987;49:741–752.

15 Majors J, Varmus HE: A small region of the mouse mammary tumor virus long terminal repeat confers glucocorticoid hormone regulation on a linked heterologous gene. Proc Natl Acad Sci USA 1983;80:5866–5870.

16 Navre M, Ringold GM: A growth factor-repressible gene associated with protein kinase C-mediated inhibition of adipocyte differentiation. J Cell Biol 1988;107:279–286.

17 Nguyen HT, Medford RM, Nadal-Ginard B: Reversibility of muscle differentiation in the absence of commitment: analysis of a myogenic cell line temperature-sensitive for commitment. Cell 1983;34:281–293.

18 Scheidereit C, Geisse S, Westphal HM, Beato M: The glucocorticoid receptor binds to defined nucleotide sequences near the promoter of mouse mammary tumor virus. Nature 1983;304:749–752.

19 Schönthal A, Herrlich P, Rahmsdorf HJ, Ponta H: Requirement for fos gene expression in the transcriptional activation of collagenase by other oncogenes and phorbol esters. Cell 1988;54:325–334.

20 Sunahara GI, Guenat C, Grieu F: Characterization of 3-methylcholanthrene effects on the rat glucocorticoid receptor in vivo. Cancer Res 1989;49:3535–3541.

21 Topper YJ, Freeman CS: Multiple hormone interactions in the developmental biology of the mammary gland. Physiol Rev 1980;60:1049–1106.

Dr. P. Herrlich, Kernforschungszentrum Karlsruhe,
Institut für Genetik und Toxikologie,
Postfach 3640, D-7500 Karlsruhe 1 (FRG)

Contrib Oncol, vol 39, pp 10–22 (Karger, Basel, 1990)

Transcription Factor-Encoding Oncogenes: The Fos/Jun Paradigm

R. Müller, F. C. Lucibello, M. Neuberg, M. Schuermann

Institut für Molekularbiologie und Tumorforschung (IMT),
Philipps-Universtität Marburg, Marburg, FRG

A great number of results obtained within the last two years has provided overwhelming evidence that Fos plays a pivotal role in the regulation of transcription (for a review see [1]). Following the observation that c-Fos is present in a transcription complex bound to the promoter of the gene encoding the adipocyte protein -2 (aP2) [2] it could be demonstrated that the Fos protein complex binds to the DNA recognition sequence (TRE) of the transcription factor AP1 [3 – 8]. AP1 had previously been identified by virtue of its sequence-specific interaction with the SV40 early promoter region and its inducibility by the tumor promoter TPA [9 – 11]. A major component of AP1 is the product of the protooncogene c-*jun* [12, 13], which in turn is part of the previously identified Fos-associated p39 proteins, pointing to a functional interaction between the two nuclear proto-oncogene products [3, 5, 7, 14 – 17]. In agreement with these observations it could be shown that Fos is able to transactivate AP1 dependent transcription in transient assays where Fos expression vectors were cotransferred with a chimeric TRE-HSVtk promoter-CAT construct into different cell lines [5, 7, 8, 21]. In addition, Fos has also transrepressing properties and can downregulate transcription of the c-fos promoter [6, 18 – 20].

The formation of a Fos/Jun complex is a prerequisite for high affinity binding to the AP1 binding site (TRE) [21 – 25]. The affinity of a c-Fos/c-Jun complex is at least 30-fold higher than that of a c-Jun homodimer and c-Fos is unable to bind at all due to its failure to homodimerize [22]. This suggests that at least one function of Fos is to increase the affinity of Jun for the TRE through cooperative binding and/or vice versa.

Despite our increasing knowledge of the molecular properties of the c-Fos protein we are far from understanding the mechanism by which Fos transforms a cell. In fibroblasts and other mesenchymal cells, which represent the target cells for transformation by Fos, the endogenous c-*fos* gene is subject to stringent control mechanisms and only transiently induced by growth factor signals [26–28]. On the other hand the normal c-Fos protein possesses transforming properties; structural alterations in the regulatory upstream elements and the RNA destabilizing 3'-non-coding region suffice to activate the transforming potential of c-*fos* [29–31]. Additional alterations in the coding region, as they occur in the viral *fos* genes, only have an enhancing effect on the transforming potential [29, 32]. It has therefore been postulated that the induction of transformation by Fos protein is a consequence of its deregulated expression. The transformation-revelant cellular targets of Fos, however, are unknown. Likewise, it is not clear which of the known molecular properties of Fos are relevant for the induction of transformation, e.g. whether transrepression plays a pivotal role in transformation as in the case of the adenovirus E1a oncogene [33]. To address this question and to elucidate the mechanism of transrepression we have undertaken a structure-function analysis of the mouse c-*fos* promoter and the Fos protein. Here, we give a summary of the results obtained so far. Our observations suggest a correlation between Fos/Jun binding complex formation, interaction with the TRE and transactivation, but not transrepression.

The Leucine Repeat Motif in Fos is the Jun Binding Site and is Required for Transformation

In the first part of this study we intended to determine the approximate location of the p39 binding site in Fos by immunoprecipitation of terminally truncated Fos proteins. Previously performed deletion analyses had shown that truncated Fos proteins were coprecipitated with p39 jun as long as a region in the middle of Fos (amino acids 171–220) was present. This highly conserved region [34] contains a motif described by Landschulz et al. [35] as a structure common to a subclass of DNA binding proteins including Fos, Jun, MYC and C/EBP. This motif consists of a periodic repetition (4–5) of leucines at every 7th position in a predicted α-helical structure over a distance of at least 8 helical turns. In an idealized α-helix the leucine residues would thus lie on one side of the helix. The side chain of the leucine residues extending from the helix of one protein could thus form hydrophobic bonds with the leucine side chains of the helix from another protein containing a similar structure. The results of a detailed structure-function analysis are consistent with the model proposed by Landschulz et al. [35] for the interaction between Fos and Jun. Mutagenesis of single or multiple leucine residues in Fos had distinct effects on the ability of the resultant proteins to form complexes with Jun. The binding properties of the mutant Fos proteins could be quantitated as follows:

Fos wild type $\cong$ L3 > L4, L5, L2 > L1, L3 - L4 > L1 - L4 $\geq$ L2 - L4, L4 - L5, L3 - L4 - L5 $\cong$ 0 % binding.

According to these results it appears that all of the five leucines participate in the interaction with Jun, but that the different leucine residues have different functional importance. Mutagenesis of the third leucine (Leu-179) had the least pronounced effect, in the mutant protein containing a single change (L3) as well as in the double mutant L3 - L4. The reason for this may be its location in the middle of the 'zipper' so that its absence may be compensated for by the adjacent leucines. The validity of the 'leucine zipper' model is further substantiated by an observation predicted by hypothetical consideration: Impairment of the orientation of the leucine residues on one side of the helix by insertion of additional amino acids between two leucine residues (FA183ins) practically abolishes binding to Jun.

Similar results on the relevance of leucine residues for Fos/Jun complex formation have been reported by several other groups [23, 36 - 38]. More recent studies strongly suggest that other amino acid interactions are also crucial for the formation of a stable Fos/Jun complex, and probably determine the specificity of interaction (M. S. and R. M., unpublished observations). These include those amino acids which, in the arrangement of an ideal α-helix, are located adjacent to the leucine residues (i. e., amino acids in positions 1, 3 and 4 relative to the preceding leucine). In addition, our results suggest that His-200 (marked by a dot in figure 1) which is conserved in all Fos and Jun proteins is crucial for complex formation. The precise nature of these interactions between positions 1, 3 and 4, however, remains to be investigated. A model of the Fos/Jun leucine zipper is shown in figure 1. Hydrophobic bonds between leucines are indicated by dotted lines and amino acids in other critical positions are marked by underlining (position 1), boxes (position 3) or circles (position 4).

Our data also clearly indicate a strong correlation between the Jun binding and transforming potential of the mutant Fos proteins. This suggests that the presence of a functional leucine repeat structure that is able to mediate interaction with other proteins containing a similar binding site such as the one in Jun is indispensable for the induction of transformation.

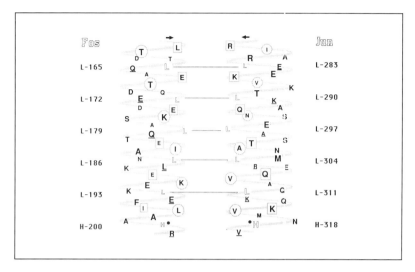

Fig. 1. Model of the Fos/Jun leucine zipper. The figure shows the arrangement of amino acids in an ideal α-helix. Arrows indicate direction (N → C-terminus), dotted lines show interactions between leucines. Amino acids in position 1 are underlined, in position 3 boxed and in position 4 circled. The histidine residues in Fos and Jun which are crucial for their interaction are marked with a dot.

Two Functionally Different Regions in Fos are Required for the Sequence-Specific DNA Interaction of the Fos/Jun Protein Complex

We next attempted to identify two regions in Fos which are required for binding the complex to the TRE. We concentrated this investigation on the middle region of Fos, which evolutionarily is the most highly conserved [34] and is crucial for the induction of transformation [32] and transactivation [8]. Two long α-helical regions are predicted in this region, the leucine zipper between amino acids 163–202 and a basic region between positions 139–156 [39]. In addition to the leucine zipper mutants described above, various mutants altered in the first helix by exchanging single, pairs or triplets of basic amino acids either with other basic (Arg → Lys; Lys → Arg) or with neutral (Arg, Lys → Gln) amino acids by altering the non-polar sequence Met-Ala-Ala-Ala were analyzed in band shift assays for their potential to form a Fos/Jun/TRE complex. As expected, the ability of the leucine-repeat mutants (L3, L4, L2, L3–4–5, FA183ins) to form a stable Fos/Jun/DNA complex correlated well with their ability to associate with Jun [40]: the substitution of Leu 179 (L3), Leu 183 (L4) or Leu 172 (L2) either did not affect (L3) or decreased (L4; L2) the Fos/Jun/DNA complex formation, whereas the triple leucine mutants L3–4–5 and the insertion mutants FA183ins, in which the orientation of leucine resides on one side of the helix is impaired, did not allow complex formation to any significant extent. These data indicate that the association of Fos and Jun through the leucine zipper is required for their interaction with the AP1 DNA-recognition sequence.

Gel retardation analysis of the other mutant Fos proteins revealed that the basic α-helical domain in Fos is also involved in Fos/Jun/DNA complex formation, as indicated by the reduced ability of mutant D9 and the failure of D3, D15, D19 ins, D4 and D16 to form a Fos/Jun/DNA complex. Three aspects of these results deserve particular attention. First, there is no correlation between the elimination of positive charges and the impairment of binding. D6 and D8 (three and two basic amino acids replaced with glutamine, respectively) showed either no change or only a small reduction in their complex-forming potential. In contrast, the mutants having basic for basic amino-acid substitutions (D16) or an altered hydrophobic stretch (D15, D19 ins) completely lost their complex-forming potential. Second, the results suggest that specific interactions with DNA occur in this Fos domain. Although the alteration of certain pairs or triplets of amino acids (D6, D7) did not affect DNA binding ability, the substitution of a single amino acid in D9 or the double mutation in D16 led to a reduction or the abrogation of DNA complex formation. Third, those sequences identified here as being crucial for the formation of a stable Fos/Jun/DNA complex are identical with those most highly conserved between Fos and Jun, namely the putative DNA-binding site in Jun [41].

Because Fos cannot form a homodimer it could not be directly analysed whether Fos specifically recognizes part of the TRE or has a different role in the binding of the Fos-Jun complex to DNA. To engineer a recombinant Fos protein that was able to form a homodimeric DNA-binding site we exchanged the leucine zipper in Fos with that of Jun. This ψ-Fos protein could indeed be shown to form a pseudo-homodimer with Fos in an in vitro complex-reconstitution assay [25]. This demonstrates that it is the structure of the leucine zipper that normally prevents the formation of Fos homodimers and suggests that amino acids other than leucines play a crucial role in the interaction. When Fos, ψ-Fos and Jun proteins were analyzed in a comparative band shift assay the following results were obtained: (1) Under the conditions used no binding was observed with Fos or Jun alone, but the Fos-Jun complex bound cooperatively. Under different experimental conditions, that is if the concentration of Jun protein or oligonucleotide probe is increased, it is possible to detect low affinity of binding of Jun homodimers; (2) the Fos ψ-Fos complex efficiently bound to the TRE oligonucleotide; and (3) both the ψ-Fos homodimer and a ψ-Fos-Jun heterodimer also bound to the TRE oligonucleotide, but with less affinity than the Fos-ψ-Fos complex. These results demonstrate that the DNA-binding site of Fos can interact specifically with the TRE provided that a dimeric complex is formed. It is likely that in the natural Fos-Jun complex the situation is similar. Our observations, therefore support the hypothesis that Fos and Jun interact with one half site of the TRE each. The TRE, however, as shown by UV-crosslinking and mutagenesis of the TRE [42] is not perfectly symmetrical. This might explain why a Fos/Jun complex binds with higher affinity to the TRE that an Fos/ψ-Fos complex.

Transrepression of the Mouse c-fos Promoters: A Novel Mechanism of Fos-Mediated Transregulation

C-Fos protein has also been reported to possess transrepressing properties in that it has a negative regulatory effect on the human c-*fos* and heat shock protein 70 (HSP70) promoters [18, 43, 44]. Multiple regulatory sites in the c-*fos* promoter have been identified, most notably the serum response element (SRE), which is the major mediator of growth factor stimulation and represents a binding site for different proteins or protein complexes [45 – 57]. Another binding site for a growth factor inducible protein complex of unknown nature and function has been described ~40 nucleotides upstream of the SRE [58]. In addition, there is a binding site for AP1 (TRE) directly adjacent to the SRE [43, 44, 59, 60] and at least one cyclic AMP responsive element (CRE) at position -60 [43, 61 – 63].

Analysis of c-*fos*-CAT constructs, where individual or several of TRE and ATF sites were mutated or deleted, showed only a slightly reduced repression by Fos compared to constructs containing the intact c-*fos* upstream region. This applies even to a construct consisting of just the SRE fused to mouse c-*fos* upstream sequences starting at position – 46, i. e., the TATA box plus 11 adjacent nucleotides. These observations strongly suggest that the SRE itself rather than any of the TRE, CRE or other structurally related elements is the major target of repression. To clarify whether several elements may cooperate in repression of the mouse c-*fos* promoter we performed titration experiments. Increasing amounts of the Fos expression vector were cotransfected with different c-*fos*-CAT plasmids to determine the amount of Fos required for half maximum repression in the absence or presence of different regulatory elements in the c-*fos* promoter. If two elements cooperated, e.g., the SRE with a TRE, one would expect that more Fos protein is required for half maximum repression if one of the elements is deleted. However, the results argue against such a possibility, since similar values were obtained regardless of the presence or absence of the TRE, CRE or potential ATF sites. Interestingly, in addition to its function in mediating induction by the tumor promoter TPA [60] the TRE seems to play a role in the regulation of basal level activity in that it decreases basal promoter activity [19, 20]. It may depend on the precise composition and/or modification (e.g. by TPA-induced phosphorylation), of the protein complex binding to the TRE whether a repressing or an activating effect is achieved. Similar observations have recently been made with the human c-*fos* promoter by König et al. [19].

When a series of mutated Fos proteins were analyzed for their transrepressing potential another unexpected observation was made. Fos proteins defective in DNA (TRE) binding are able to transrepress, in some cases even more efficiently than the unaltered Fos protein. This finding is in agreement with the results discussed above, i.e., the fact that the TRE or related elements do not play a crucial role in the repression of serum induction. One could speculate that transrepression may involve the interaction of Fos with (an) other regulatory site(s). This seems, however, to be rather unlikely, considering that even a mutant like D19 is able to transrepress efficiently. D19 contains an insertion of two alanines within the DNA binding site [25] which presumably alters the two-dimensional structure of this domain and would therefore be expected to destroy any specific interaction occurring in this region.

On the other hand, the leucine zipper seems to play an important role in transrepression, since mutants like L1–4 or L3–4–5 are unable to transrepress. This suggests that Fos must form a complex with another protein to be able to transrepress. It is unlikely that the SRF itself forms such a complex since it does not contain a leucine zipper [53]. Formation of such protein complexes could modify preexisting transcription complexes interacting with the SRE which are known to consist of multiple individual proteins [47, 54, 56]. Any of these components could be a direct or indirect target of Fos-mediated repression. Such protein complexes mediating the repression of serum induction could occur without additional DNA contacts being established by Fos protein. This would be in agreement with *in vivo* footprint experiments which indicate that the protein-DNA contacts in the region around the SRE do not change after transcriptional shut-down of the c-fos promoter [57].

These results discussed above clearly suggest that Fos-mediated transrepression of the mouse c-*fos* promoter is mechanistically different from the known transregulatory function of Fos protein, i. e., the transactivation of AP1 dependent transcription. First, transrepression does not require any TRE or related element in the Fos promoter, and second, Fos protein mutants defective in DNA binding are able to transrepress efficiently. It can, therefore, also be excluded that a Fos/Jun complex acts indirectly via a TRE in another gene whose product then transrepresses serum induction of c-*fos* (Tab. 1).

Conclusions

The availability of mutant Fos proteins differing in their transrepressing potential and other biochemical properties made it possible to investigate whether correlations exist between these molecular functions and transformation. Our results show that the presence of a functional leucine zipper is a prerequisite for transformation and point to another correlation, namely between DNA (TRE) binding and transformation. On the other hand, our results strongly suggest that transrepression does not correlate with transformation. Fos proteins impaired in DNA binding are able to transrepress but are defective in transformation, and v-Fos, which is unable to repress, is a potent transforming protein. These observations rule out that transrepression of the type investigated here plays a crucial role in transformation. Other transrepressing mechanisms may exist, but there is no evidence for this at present. On the other hand, transactivation shows a much better correlation with transformation, in that mutations affecting DNA (TRE) binding of Fos and consequently activation of AP1 dependent transcription also impair the transforming potential of Fos. It is therefore not unlikely that Fos-induced transformation involves the transactivation of target genes via TREs in their promoter regions. To elucidate this question further, however, it will be necessary to learn more about the mechanism of Fos-mediated transactivation, especially to identify a potential transactivating domain in Fos which could then be subjected to a detailed structure-function analysis.

Table 1. Properties of Fos-proteins mutated in the leucine zipper or the adjacent basic region

Mutant	Mutated amino acid(s)	Substituted with	Binding to Jun	Binding to TRE	TA	TR	TF
E300 (wild type)	—	—	+++	+++	+	+	++
FBJ	C-terminal frameshift		+++	ND	ND	ND	++
Leucine zipper							
L1	Leu-165	Val	+	ND	−	ND	±
L2	Leu-172	Val	++	ND	+	ND	±
L3	Leu-179	Val	+++	++	+	+	++
L4	Leu-186	Ale	++	ND	+	ND	++
L5	Leu-193	Val	++	ND	+	ND	++
L1-L4	Leu-165, Leu 186	Val, Ala	−	−	−	−	−
L2-L4	Leu 172, Leu 186	Val, Ala	−	ND	ND	ND	−
L3-L4	Leu-179, Leu 186	Val, Ala	±	ND	ND	ND	−
L4-L5	Leu-186, Leu 193	Ala, Val		ND	ND	ND	−
L3-L4-L5	Leu 179, Leu 186, Leu 193	Val, Ala, Val	−	−	−	−	±
FA183ins	ins at pos. 183	Phe + Ala	−	−	−	ND	−
Basic region							
D13	Arg-143, Arg-144	Lys, Lys	+++	+++	ND	+	−
D8	Arg-146, Lys-148	Gln, Gln	+++	++	ND	+	++
D9	Lys-148	Gln	+++	+	ND	ND	−
D15	Met-149, Ale-150, Ala-151, Ala-152	Leu, Ser, Ser, Ser	+++	−	−	ND	−
D19	ins at pos. 151	Ala + Ala	+++	−	−	+	−
D16	Lys-153, Arg-155	Arg, Lys	+++	−	−	+	−
D17	Arg-157, Arg-158, Arg-159	Lys, Lys, Ls	+++	++++	+	++	++

TA: Transactivation, TR: Transrepression, TF: Transformation (Indication of Foci on 208F cells),
ND: not done

References

1 Curran T, Franza BRJ: Fos and Jun: The AP-1 connection. Cell 1988;55:395–397.
2 Distel RJ, Ro HS, Rosen BS, et al: Nucleoprotein complexes that regulate gene expresion in adipocyte differentiation: direct participation of c-*fos*. Cell 1987;49:835–844.
3 Rauscher III FJ, Sambucetti LC, Curran T, et al: A common DNA binding site for Fos protein complexes and transcription factor AP-1. Cell 1988;52:471–480.

4   Franza Jr BR, Rauscher III FJ, Josephs SF, et al: The *fos* complex and *fos*-related antigens recognize sequence elements that contain AP-1 binding sites. Science 1988; 239:1150–1153.

5   Sassone-Corsi P, Lamph WW, Kamps M, et al: *Fos*-associated cellular p39 is related to nuclear transcription factor AP-1. Cell 1988;54:553–560.

6   Sassone-Corsi P, Ransone LJ, Lamph WW, et al: Direct interaction between fos and jun nuclear oncoproteins: role of the 'leucine zipper' domain. Nature 1988;336: 692–695.

7   Chiu R, Boyle WJ, Meek J, et al: The c-Fos protein interacts with c-Jun/AP-1 to stimulate transcription of AP-1 responsive genes. Cell 1988;54:541–552.

8   Lucibello FC, Neuberg M, Hunter JB, et al: Transactivation of gene expression by fos protein: involvement of a binding site for the transcription factor AP-1. Oncogene 1988;3:43–51.

9   Angel P, Imagawa M, Chiu R, et al: Phorbol ester-inducible genes contain a common *cis* element recognized by a TPA-modulated *trans*-acting factor. Cell 1987;49:729–739.

10 Lee W, Mitchell P, Tjian R: Purified transcription factor AP-1 interacts with TPA-inducible enhancer elements. Cell 1987;49:741–752.

11 Jones NC, Rigby PW, Ziff EB: *Trans*-acting protein factors and the regulation of eukaryotic transcription: lessons from studies on DNA tumor viruses. Genes Dev 1988;2:267–281.

12 Bohmann D, Bos TJ, Admon A, et al: Human proto-oncogene c-*jun* encodes a DNA-binding protein with structural and functional properties of transcription factor AP-1. Science 1987;238:1386–1392.

13 Angel P, Allegretto EA, Okino ST, et al: The *jun* oncogene encodes a sequence-specific transactivator similar to AP-1. Nature 1988;332:166–171.

14 Curran T, Teich NM: Identification of a 39,000-dalton protein in cells transformed by the FBJ murine osteosarcoma virus. Virol 1982;116:221–235.

15 Curran T, Van Beveren C, Ling N, et al: Viral and cellular *fos* proteins are complexed with a 39,000-dalton cellular protein. Mol Cell Biol 1985;5:167–172.

16 Franza Jr BR, Sambucetti LC, Cohen DR, et al: Analysis of *fos* protein complexes and *fos*-related antigens by high-resolution two-dimensional gel electrophoresis. Oncogene 1987;1:213–221.

17 Müller R, Bravo R, Müller D, et al: Different types of modification in c-*fos* and its associated protein p39: modulation of DNA binding by phosphorylation. Oncogene Res 1987;2:19–32.

18 Schönthal A, Herrlich P, Rahmsdorf HJ, et al: Requirement for *fos* gene expression in the transcriptional activation of collagenase by other oncogenes and phorbol esters. Cell 1988;54:325–334.

19 König H, Ponta H, Rahmsdorf U, et al: Autoregulation of fos: the dyad symmetry elements as the major target of repression. EMBO J 89;8:2559–2566.

20 Lucibello FC, Lowag C, Neuberg M, et al: *Trans*-repression of the mouse c-*fos* promoters: a novel mechanism of Fos-mediated *trans*-regulation. Cell 1989;59:999–1007.

21 Nakabeppu Y, Ryder K, Nathans D: DNA binding activity of three murine Jun proteins: stimulation by Fos. Cell 1988;55:907–915.

22   Halazonetis TD, Georgopoulos K, Greenberg ME, et al: c-Jun dimerizes with itself
      and with c-Fos, forming complexes of different DNA binding affinities. Cell 1988;
      55:917–924.

23   Kouzarides T, Ziff E: The role of the leucine zipper in the fos-jun interaction. Nature
      1988;36:646–651.

24   Rauscher III FJ, Voulalas PJ, Franza RJ, et al: Fos and Jun bind cooperatively to the
      AP-1 site: reconstitution in vitro. Genes Dev 1988;2:1687–1699.

25   Neuberg M, Schuerman M, Hunter JB, et al: Two funtionally different regions in Fos
      are required for the sequence-specific DNA interaction of the Fos/Jun protein
      complex. Nature 1989;338:589–590.

26   Greenberg ME, Ziff EB, et al: Stimulation of 3T3 cells induces transcription of the
      c-*fos* proto-oncogene. Nature 1984;311:433–438.

27   Müller R, Bravo R, Burckhardt J, et al: Induction of c-*fos* gene and protein by growth
      factors precedes activation of c-*myc*. Nature 1984;312:716–720.

28   Kruijer W, Cooper JA, Hunter T, et al: Platelet-derived growth factor induces rapid
      but transient expression of the c-*fos* gene and protein. Nature 1984;312:711–716.

29   Miller AD, Curran T, Verma IM: c-*fos* protein can induce cellular transformation:
      a novel mechanism of activation of a cellular oncogene. Cell 1984;36:51–60.

30   Meijlink F, Curran T, Miller AD, et al: Removal of a 67-base-pair sequence in the
      noncoding region of protooncogene *fos* converts it to a transforming gene. Proc Natl
      Acad Sci USA 1985;82:4987–4991.

31   Wilson T, Treisman R: Fos C-terminal mutations block down-regulation of c-*fos*
      transcription following serum-stimulation. EMBO J 1988;7:4193–4202.

32   Jenuwein T, Müller R: Structure-function analysis of *fos* protein: a single amino acid
      change activates the immortalizing potential of v-*fos*. Cell 1987;48:647–657.

33   Lillie JW, Green M, Green MR: An adenovirus E1a protein region required for trans-
      formation and transcriptional repression. Cell 1986;46:1043–1051.

34   Mölders H, Jenuwein T, Adamkiewicz J, et al: Isolation and structural analysis of a
      biologically active chicken c-*fos* cDNA: identification of evolutionarily conserved
      domains in *fos* protein. Oncogene 1987;1:377–385.

35   Landschulz WH, Johnson PF, McKnight SL: The leucine zipper: a hypothetical struc-
      ture common to a new class of DNA binding proteins. Science 1988;240:1759–1764.

36   Gentz R, Rauscher III FJ, Abate C, et al: Parallel association of Fos and Jun leucine
      zippers juxtaposes DNA binding domains. Science 1989;243:1695–1699.

37   Turner R, Tjian R: Leucine repeats and an adjacent DNA binding domain mediate
      the formation of functional cFos-cJun heterodimers. Science 1989;243:1689–1694.

38   Ransone LJ, Visvader J, Sassone-Corsi P, et al: Fos-Jun interaction: mutational
      analysis of the leucine zipper domain of both proteins. Genes Dev 1989;3:770–781.

39   Vingron M, Nordheim A, Müller R: Anatomy of *fos* proteins. Oncogene Res 1988;
      3:1–7.

40   Schuermann M, Neuberg M, Hunter JB, et al: The leucine repeat motif in Fos protein
      mediates complex formation with Jun/AP1 and is required for transformation. Cell
      1989;56:597–516.

41   Vogt PK, Bos TJ, Doolittle RF: Homology between the DNA-binding domain of the
      GCN4 regulatory protein of yeast and the carboxyl-terminal region of a protein
      coded for by the oncogene jun. Proc Natl Acad Sci USA 1987;84:3316–3319.

42   Risse G, Jooss K, Neuberg M, et al: Asymmetrical recognition of the structurally sym-
      metrical AP1 binding site (TRE) by the Fos/Jun complex. EMBO J 1989;8:3825–3832.
43   Schönthal A, Büscher M, Angel P, et al: The Fos and Jun/Ap-1 proteins are involved
      in the downregulation of Fos transcription. Oncogene 1989;4:629–636.
44   Sassone-Corsi P, Sisson JC, Verma IM: Transcriptional autoregulation of the proto-
      oncogene *fos*. Nature 1988;334:314–319.
45   Treisman R: Transient accumulation of c-*fos* RNA following serum stimulation
      requires a conserved 5'-element and c-*fos* 3' seqences. Cell 1985;42:889–902.
46   Treisman R: Identification of a protein-binding site that mediates transcriptional
      response of the c-*fos* gene to serum factors. Cell 1986;46:567–574.
47   Treisman R: Identification and purification of a polypeptide that binds to the c-*fos*
      serum response element. EMBO J 1987;6:2711–2717.
48   Deschamps J, Meijlink F, Verma IM: Identification of a transcriptional enhancer ele-
      ment upstream from the proto-oncogene *fos*. Science 1985;230:1174–1177.
49   Prywes R, Roeder RG: Inducible binding of a factor to the c-*fos* enhancer. Cell 1986;
      47:777–784.
50   Prywes R, Roeder RG: Purification of the c-*fos* enhancer-binding protein. Mol Cell
      Biol 1987;7:3482–3489.
51   Gilman MZ, Wilson RN, Weinberg RA: Multiple protein-binding sites in the 5'-
      flanking region regulate c-*fos* expression. Mol Cell Biol 1986;6:4305–4316.
52   Greenberg ME, Siegfried Z, Ziff EB: Mutation of the c-*fos* gene dyad symmetry
      element inhibits serum inducibility of transcription in vivo and the nuclear regulatory
      factor binding in vitro. Mol Cell Biol 1987;7:1217–1225.
53   Norman C, Runswick M, Pollock R, et al: Isolation and properties of cDNA clones
      encoding SRF, a transcription factor that binds to the c-*fos* serum response element.
      Cell 1988;55:989–1003.
54   Ryan WA Jr, Franza BR Jr, Gilman MZ: Two distinct cellular phosphoproteins bind
      to the c-*fos* serum response element. EMBO J 1989;8:1785–1792.
55   Siegfried Z, Ziff EB: Transcription activation by serum, PDGF, and TPA through the
      c-*fos* DSE: Cell type specific requirements for induction. Oncogene 1989;4:3–11.
56   Shaw PE, Schröter H, Nordheim A: The ability of a ternary complex to form over the
      serum response element correlates with serum inducibility of the human c-*fos* pro-
      moter. Cell 1989;56:563–572.
57   Herrera RE, Shaw PE, Nordheim A: Occupation of the c-*fos* serum response element
      in vivo by a multi-protein complex is unaltered by growth factor induction. Nature
      1989;340:68–70.
58   Hayes TE, Kitchen AM, Cochran BH: Inducible binding of a factor to the c-*fos*
      regulatory region. Proc Natl Acad Sci USA 1987;84:1272–1276.
59   Piette J, Yaniv M: Two different factors bind to the α-domain of the polyoma virus
      enhancer, one of which also interacts with the SV-40 and c-*fos* enhancers. EMBO J
      1987;6:1331–1337.
60   Fisch TM, Prywes R, Roeder G: An AP1 binding site in the c-fos gene can mediate
      induction by epidermal growth factor and 12-*O*-tetradecanoyl phorbol-13-acetate.
      Mol Cell Biol 1989;9:1327–1331.
61   Sassone-Corsi P, Visvader J, Ferland L, et al: Induction of proto-oncogene *fos* tran-
      scription through the adenylate cyclase pathway: characterization of a cAMP-respon-
      sive element. Genes Dev 1988;2:1529–1538.

62   Büscher M, Rahmsdorf HJ, Litfin M, et al: Activation of the c-*fos* gene by UV and
     phorbol ester: different signal transduction pathways converge to the same enhancer
     element. Oncogene 1988;3:301–311.
63   Fisch TM, Prywes R, Simon MC, et al: Multiple sequences element in the c-*fos*
     promoter mediate induction by cAMP. Genes Dev 1989;3:198–211.

R. Müller, Institut für Molekularbiologie und Tumorforschung (IMT),
Philipps-Universität Marburg,
Emil-Mannkopff-Straße 2, D-3550 Marburg (FRG)

Contrib Oncol, vol 39, pp 23–34 (Karger, Basel, 1990)

Casein Kinase II is Involved in the Regulation of Several Nuclear Oncoproteins

B. Lüscher, R. N. Eisenman

Fred Hutchinson Cancer Research Center, Seattle, WA, USA

The identification of retroviral oncogenes and their cellular homologes (protooncogenes) has made it possible to study a set of genes implicated in the regulation of cell growth and differentiation. The protein products of a subset of these (proto)oncogenes are localized to the cell nucleus. Recent studies have revealed that at least several of these nuclear oncoproteins (Fos, Jun, Myb, Erb A) are directly involved in the regulation of gene expression by binding to response elements in the promoter region of genes modulating gene transcription [4, 18, 29, 40]. A prediction from these data would be that these oncoproteins are involved in the positive or negative regulation of genes which promote cell growth and/or cell differentiation. In addition to these cell derived sequences the products of oncogenes of several DNA tumor viruses such as large T antigen of SV40, E1A of Adenovirus and E7 of human papillomavirus are localized in the nucleus. Multiple functions have been assigned to these gene products. One of the potentially important steps in the ability to alter growth properties of cells is their interaction with the retinoblastoma gene product (Rb) [6]. Several lines of evidence suggest that Rb functions as an antioncogene, inhibiting cell growth in its active form. It is hypothesized that the interaction of large T antigen (T ag), E1A and E7 with Rb abolishes Rb's function thus depriving cells of a crucial mechanism to negatively regulate cell growth.

The short term regulation of these oncoproteins in response to various signals seems to be desirable to adjust cellular growth and/or differentiation to an altered environment. There are at least two possible ways of how short term regulation could be achieved. First many of these nuclear oncoproteins appear to have a short half-life allowing rapid up or down regulation of their amounts. This has been observed for porteins such as Fos and Myc when cells in Go are stimulated to enter the cell cycle. In addition Myc levels are rapidly down regulated when HL-60 cells are induced to differentiate (for a review see [11]). Second, all of these nuclear oncoproteins are modified by phosphorylation. Phosphorylation is a major mechanism by which the cell can reversibly modify proteins and thus potentially modulate their activity (for a review see [10]). In a search for possible phosphorylation consensus sequences, we determined that all nuclear oncoproteins analyzed contained consensus sites for casein kinase II (CKII). CKII is a Ser/Thr specific kinase which has been found to localize to both the cytoplasm and the nucleus [16, 19]. Recent evidence suggests that CKII kinase activity is modulated in response to growth factor treatment [1, 5, 17, 34]. Therefore is is conveivable that CKII could be involved in the regulation of several nuclear oncoproteins playing key roles in determining aspects of cell growth and differentiation. We have shown that several of the nuclear acting oncoproteins are substrates for CKII and that these CKII phosphorylation sites are functionally relevant [13, 19, 22, 23].

Results

CKII possesses a rather unique substrate specificity, characterized using both synthetic peptides and proteins as substrates, requiring a Ser or Thr residue in the vicinity of acidic amino acids (reviewed in [19]). It appears that the requirement for an Asp or Glu residue at position +3 relative to the acceptor Ser/Thr is most critical. Interestingly, a phosphorylated Ser or Thr residue at the +3 position can also serve as a recognition site. Acidic residues at positions +4 and +5 are second most important and acidic amino acids N-terminal to the acceptor Ser/Thr and at position +1 and +2 are favorable for CKII phosphorylation. Using model CKII consensus sequences in a computer assisted database search we identified about 350 proteins containing possible CKII phosphorylation sites. Among those were several proteins known to be phosphorylated by CKII in vitro. Most interesting was the identification of many nuclear oncoproteins as potential CKII substrates (table 1). This prompted us to test if any of these proteins would be substrates for purified CKII in vitro. We have found that Myc, Myb, Erb A, T ag and HPV E7, but not Fos, are CKII substrates.

Myc

Two regions in the Myc protein were identified as containing CKII consensus sequences: the acidic domain overlapping the exon 2/3 border

Table 1. Identification of casein kinase II substrate consensus sequences within nuclear oncoproteins

Protein	Sequence	Reference
Ck-Myc*	$P_{222}PTTSSDSEEEQEEDEE_{238}$ $E_{246}ANESESSTESSTEASEE_{263}$ $P_{322}RTSDSEENDKR_{333}$	[39]
Hu-Myc	$P_{245}PTTSSDSEEEQEDEEE_{261}$ $T_{343}SPRSSDTEENV_{354}$	[41]
Hu-N-Myc	$W_{80}GSPAEEDAF_{89}$ $L_{244}STSGEDTLSDSDDEDDEEEDEEEE_{268}$ $R_{365}NSDSEDSERRR_{376}$	[35]
Hu-L-Myc	$C_{156}SGSESPSDSENEEI_{170}$ $P_{272}VSSDTEDV_{280}$	[20]
Ck-Myb	$R_{6}HSIYSSDDDDEDVE_{20}$ $K_{143}KTSWTEEED_{152}$ $P_{578}VSEEEGS_{585}$	[14]
Dr-Myb	$N_{14}YGSNSDSEESEYSENED_{31}$ $T_{189}AWTEKEDE_{197}$	[27]
Ck-Erb A	$P_{10}LSEPEDTR_{18}$ $P_{42}SYLDKDEQ_{50}$ $P_{156}SPSAEEWEL_{165}$ $P_{198}MASMPDGDL_{207}$	[32]
Mu-Fos	$V_{129}EQLSPEEEEKRRIRR_{144}$ $P_{228}EASTPESEEAF_{239}$	[37]
Hu-Jun	$P_{250}LSPIDMESQ_{259}$	[4]
v-Ets**	$A_{208}SSCCEDP_{215}$ $L_{590}SDPDEVA_{597}$	[26]
HPV16 E7	$L_{28}NDSSEEEDEID_{39}$	[33]
SV40 large T	$E_{107}MPSSDDEAT_{116}$ $R_{630}NSDDDDEDSQEN_{642}$	[12]
Ad 5 E1A (13S)	$P_{130}PSDDEDEEGEE_{141}$ $P_{186}VSEPEPEPEPEP_{200}$	[38]

The underlined amino acids identify possible acceptor sites for CKII.

*Ck: chicken; Hu: human; Dr: drosophiea; Mu: murine; v: viral; HPV16: human papillomavirus type 16; SV40: simian virus 40; AD 5: adeno virus type 5.

**For v-Ets, the amino acids contained in the 2.46 kb EcoR1 fragment were numbered 1–669 [26].

and the C-terminal domain (see table 1 for details). By comparative mapping using in vivo phosphorylated Myb and in vitro CKII phosphorylated Myc, or peptides spanning the CKII consensus sequences of the proteins, all the potential CKII sites were found to be phosphorylated both in vivo and in vitro by CKII [22]. At present it is not clear if CKII is an authentic Myc phosphorylating kinase or if another kinase with very similar specificity is responsible for phosphorylating the sites in vivo. The C-terminal phosphorylation site (hu-Myc$^{343-354}$) is of particular interest, as it is located just N-terminal to a region of the protein which is composed of a basic region, a helix-loop-helix domain and a leucine zipper [25, 28]. The HLH domain and the LZ have been found to be the structures dictating dimer and tetramer formation of Myc in vitro [9]. The basic region, by homology with similar regions in several DNA binding proteins, is implicated in directing sequence specific DNA binding. However, no such activity for Myc has been described yet. Due to the close physical association of the CKII phosphorylation site with these three domains one may hypothesize that CKII phosphorylation influences oligomerization and/or DNA binding.

The central CKII phosphorylation site lies in an extensive acidic region (human: residues 242–261, 10 acidic residues, 5 Ser/Thr CKII acceptor sites; chicken: residues 220–263, 18 acidic residues, 9 Ser/Thr CKII acceptor sites) implicated in macrophage and fibroblast transformation [22]. Two main roles could be envisaged for such domains. First, acidic regions in transcription factors (acid blobs) have been implicated in the interaction with RNA polymerase. Thus CKII could modulate the extent of negative charge within this region and alter interactions with the transcription machinery. Second, the acidic domain in Myc has a high PEST score [30]. PEST sequences (PEST standes for Pro, Glu, Ser, Thr rich) have been found to correlate with short protein half-lives arguing that the PEST sequences could be determinants for protein degredation. CKII phosphorylation could be read as a signal important in the regulation of the turnover rate of the Myc protein.

Myb

The analysis of the Myb nuclear oncoprotein revealed three potential CKII phosphorylation sites, the first being close to the N-terminus, the second in the DNA binding domain and the third near the C-terminus.

Various mapping procedures showed that only the site at the N-terminus was phosphorylated by CKII in vitro and that this corresponded to an authentic in vivo phosphorylation site which is highly conserved in vertebrate Myb's [23] (fig. 1). In addition, at the corresponding loccation in a Myb-related protein from Drosophila, a CKII consensus site is found despite any obvious homology in the primary sequence of the surrounding region [27]. Another interesting feature of this N-terminal phosphorylation site is its frequent deletion in almost all oncogenically activated Mybs, suggesting an important regulatory role [23].

Recent evidence strongly suggests that Myb is a bonafide transcription factor, having a DNA binding domain as well as domains regulating transcriptional activation [2, 31, 40]. Myb specifically interacts with a short DNA sequence (PyAACGG), named MRE for Myb responsive element, which is a required cis-acting element for Myb-specific transactivation. The identified CKII phosphorylation site is not contained in one of the described elements. In fact, it lies 70–80 residues upstream of the DNA binding domain, the closest of the 3 functional elements. In order to test the functional significance of the N-terminal phosphorylation site, the effect of CKII phosphorylation on the specific interaction of Myb with an MRE was tested. It was found, that CKII phosphorylation reversibly downregulated Myb DNA binding, suggesting an important modulating role of the N-terminal phosphorylation site in Myb function [23]. One prediction made from these data is, that the oncogenically activated Mybs, lacking the N-terminus, have potentially lost a negative regulatory site for DNA binding. This was confirmed by the finding that CKII had no effect on the DNA binding properties of v-Myb and N-terminal truncated c-Myb proteins. What might be the normal physiological role of CKII phosphorylation of Myb? Myb expression is mainly confined to cells in the hematopoietic system where upon terminal differentiation Myb expression is downregulated. An important concept in hematopoiesis is, that growth factor stimulation can result in both cell differentiation and cell proliferation [24]. To date, no information about the regulation of CKII activitiy in hematopoietic cells is available. However an attractive model for CKII regulation of Myb function in hematopoietic cells in response to growth factors would include a role in both the proliferative and the differentiation phases. One can envisage that genes driving cell differentiation will be turned on whereas genes involved in maintaining a certain state of differentiation and in self renewal may be, at least transiently, downregulated. CKII which is known to be growth factor modulated, could transmit signals to transiently decrease the transcription

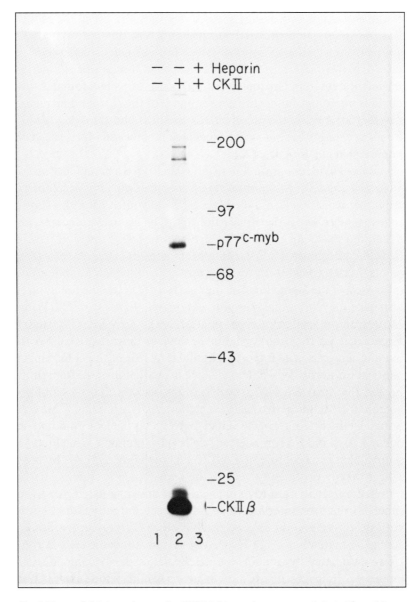

Fig. 1. Human Myb is a substrate for CKII: Myb was immunoprecipitated from Manca cells and incubated in the presence of [γ-^{32}P] ATP without CKII (lane 1), with 360 ng CKII (lane 2), or with CKII and 0.6 μM heparin (lane 3). Low doses of heparin have been found to inhibit CKII. The samples were analysed on a 10 % SDS-polyacrylamide gel (For methods, see [21, 22]).

of the latter class of genes by modulating Myb DNA binding activity. The loss of the CKII phosphorylation site in oncogenically activated Myb would render these genes nonregulatable. This in turn may lead to a population of cells frozen at a certain stage of differentiation. Such cells could be susceptible to further events leading to tumor formation. Similar conclusions have been drawn from results obtained in transgenic mice using the Eμ-myc system (for a review see [8]). Expression of Myc under the regulation of an Eμ-heavy chain enhancer in transgenic mice leads to an expanded pool of cycling pre-B cells. After a rather long latency period the animals develop clonal B cell lymphomas. These findings suggest that constitutive myc expression leads to an abnormally large population of undifferentiated pre-B cells which are targets for further activating genetic alterations leading to tumorgenic cell growth.

Erb A and Fos

Both the nuclear oncoproteins Erb A and Fos contain CKII consensus sequences (table 1). Erb A is the nuclear receptor for thyroid hormone [32]. Recently, it was found that Erb A encodes a sequence specific DNA binding protein regulating gene transcription [15, 18, 36]. To test, if Erb A could serve as a substrate for CKII in an in vitro kinase assay, Erb A was immunoprecipitated from 10T1/2 mouse fibroblasts and incubated with CKII and (γ-^{32}P) ATP. As shown in figure 2, Erb A served as a specific substrate. Four major phosphorylated proteins were detected (fig. 2 arrowheads) which is in agreement with the identification of several translation products [3]. No information as to the importance of this phosphorylation has been obtained yet.

When Fos was analyzed in a similar manner no phosphate was transfered to the immunoprecipitated Fos protein. Both CKII consensus sequences in Fos contain a Pro residue between the acceptors Ser and the +3 Glu residue. It was therefore possible, that Pro residues in such a location would be inhibitory. To test the effect of this Pro residue, a Fos[129-144] peptide (table 1) was synthesized and used in CKII kinase assays. This peptide was completely negative for CKII phosphorylation. Similarly when the basic amino acids at the C-terminal and/or the Pro was replaced by a Lys again no phosphate was transferred. However, replacing Pro with Glu was sufficient to generate a CKII substrate (B. L., E. C., R. E. unpublished observation). It was concluded that Pro and basic residues, when located at posi-

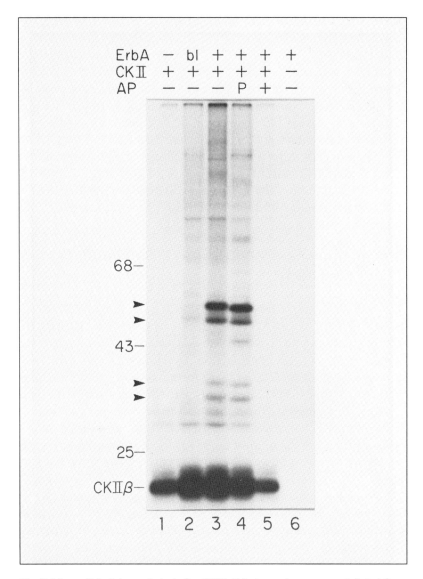

Fig. 2. Mouse Erb A is a substrate for CKII. Erb A was immunoprecipitated from mouse fibroblasts (10T1/2 cells). Erb A immunoprecipitates and CKII (360 ng) were added as indicated in the presence of [γ-^{32}P] ATP. Alkaline phosphatase (AP) treatment was performed after the CKII kinase reaction. bl: Erb A immunoprecipitation was blocked by adding excess immunogen. P: AP pretreatment of the Erb A immunocomplex prior to CKII phosphorylation. Samples were analysed on a 10 % SDS-polyacrylamide gel (For methods see [3, 22]).

tion +1 and possibly +2 to the acceptor Ser/Thr, are inhibitory of CKII phosphorylation. However, more peptides will have to be tested to define if this is true in general.

E7 and T ag

We have also analysed the CKII phosphorylation of the two DNA tumor virus encoded nuclear oncoproteins HPV16 E7 and SV40T ag [13, 19]. Both were found to be phosphorylated by CKII in vitro at authentic sites. CKII phosphorylates a subset of in vivo phosphorylation sites in T ag, whereas E7 is phosphorylated in vitro and in vivo at a single site. Interestingly the CKII phosphorylation sites in E7 and T ag, as well as a potential CKII site in E1A are proximal to the Rb binding site. An attractive possibility is, that CKII is part of the regulatory mechanism determining the interaction between these tumor antigens and Rb.

Mutational analysis of the E7 protein was used to confirm the localization of the CKII phosphorylation site and functional analysis of such mutants indicated a positive regulatory effect of CKII phosphorylation (J.F., B.L., R.E. manuscript in preparation).

Conclusions

We have concluded that all the established nuclear oncoproteins contain CKII phosphorylation consensus sequences. Several of these oncoproteins were identified as in vitro and/or in vivo substrates for CKII or a kinase with very similar specificity. The functional analysis of these CKII phosphorylation sites, as far as assayed, revealed their functional importance. For Myb phosphorylation at the CKII site modulates DNA binding. Molecules which are phosphorylated are not binding to an MRE. For Myc and HPV16 E7, mutation at the CKII sites alter their transforming capacity in cotransformation assays. Together with the described properties of CKII, such as the modulation of its activity in response to growth factors and its in part nuclear localization, make this enzyme a candidate to be an important regulator for nuclear proteins during cell growth. However, to this end, no direct correlation between a change in CKII activity and an altered function of any of the proteins described here has been established. The challenge for future experiments will be to interdigitate growth factor action, CKII activity and nuclear events such as Myb specific transcription.

Acknowledgements

We are grateful to D. Litchfield for purified CKII and J. Smith for secretarial assistance. This work was supported by grants from the National Cancer Institute (NIH) to RNE and by a postdoctoral fellowship from the Swiss National Science Foundation to BL.

References

1 Ackerman P, Osheroff N: Regulation of casein kinase II activity by epidermal growth factor in human A-431 carcinoma cells. J Biol Chem 1989;264:11958–11965.

2 Biedenkapp H, Borgmeyer U, Sippel AE, Klempnauer KH: Viral *myb* oncogene encodes a sequence-specific DNA-binding activity. Nature 1988;335:835–837.

3 Bigler J, Eisenman RN: c-*erb*A encodes multiple proteins in chicken erythroid cells. Mol Cell Biol 1988;8:4155–4161.

4 Bohmann D, Bos TJ, Admon A, Nishimura T, Vogt PK, Tijan R: Human proto-oncogene c-jun encodes a DNA binding protein with structural and functional properties of transcription factor AP-1. Science 1987;238:1386–1392.

5 Carroll D, Marshak DR: Serum stimulated cell growth causes oscillations in casein kinase II activity. J Biol Chem 1989;264:7345–7348.

6 Cooper JA, Whyte P: RB and the cell cycle: Entrance or exit? Cell 1989;58:1009–1011.

7 Corvera S, Roach PJ, DePaoli-Roach AA, Czech MP: Insulin action inhibits insulin-like growth factor-II (IGF-II) receptor phosphorylation in H-35 hepatoma cells. J Biol Chem 1988;263:3116–3122.

8 Cory S, Adams JM: Transgenic mice and oncogenesis. Ann Rev Immunol 1988;6:25–48.

9 Dang CV, McGuire M, Buckmire M, Lee WMF: Involvement of the 'leucine zipper' region in the oligomerization and transforming activity of human c-myc protein. Nature 1989;337:664–666.

10 Edelman AM, Blumenthal DA, Krebs EG: Protein serine and threonine kinases. Ann Rev Biochem 1987;56:567–613.

11 Eisenman RN, Thompson CB: Oncogenes with potential nuclear function: *myc, myb* and *fos*. Cancer Surv 1986;5:309–327.

12 Fiers W, Contreras R, Haegeman G, Rogiers R, van de Voorde A, Heuverswyn H, van Herreweghe J, Volckaert G, Ysebaert M: The total nucleotide sequence of SV40 DNA. Nature 1978;273:113–120.

13 Firzlaff JM, Galloway DA, Eisenman RN, Lüscher B: The E7 protein of human papillomavirus type 16 is phosphorylated by casein kinase II. New Biol 1989;1:44–53.

14 Gerondakis S, Bishop JM: Structure of the protein encoded by the chicken proto-oncogene c-*myb*. Mol Cell Biol 1986;6:3677–3684.

15 Glass CK, Franco R, Weinberger C, Albert VR, Evans RM, Rosenfeld MG: A c-*erb*-A binding site in rat growth hormone gene mediates *trans*-activation by thyroid hormone. Nature 1987;329:738–741.

16 Hathaway GM, Traugh JA: Casein kinases-multipotential protein kinases. Curr Top Cell Reg 1982;21:101–127.

17 Klarlund JK, Czech MP: Insulin-like growth factor I and insulin rapidly increase casein kinase II activity in BALB/c 3T3 fibroblasts. J Biol Chem 1988;263:15872–15875.

18 Koenig RJ, Brent GA, Warne RL, Larsen PR, Moore DD: Thyroid hormone receptor binds to a site in the rat growth hormone promoter required for induction by thyroid hormone. Proc Natl Acad Sci USA 1987;84:5670–5674.

19 Krebs EG, Eisenman RN, Kuenzel EA, Litchfield DW, Lozeman FJ, Lüscher B, Sommercorn J: Casein kinase II as a potentially important enzyme concerned with signal transduction. Cold Sping Harbor Symp. Quant Biol 1988;LIII:77–84.

20 Legouy E, DePinho R, Zimmerman K, Collum R, Yancopoulos G, Mitsock L, Kriz R, Alt FW: Structure and expression of the murine L-*myc* gene. EMBO J 1987;6:3359–3366.

21 Lüscher B, Eisenman RN: c-*myc* and c-*myb* protein degradation: Effect of metabolic inhibitors and heat shock. Mol Cell Biol 1988;8:2504–2512.

22 Lüscher B, Kuenzel EA, Krebs EG, Eisenman RN: Myc oncoproteins are phosphorylated by casein kinase II. EMBO J 1989;8:1111–1119.

23 Lüscher B, Christenson E, Litchfield DW, Krebs EG, Eisenman RN: Myb DNA binding is inhibited by casein kinase II phosphorylation at a site deleted during oncogenic activation. Nature 1990;344:517–522.

24 Metcalf D: The molecular control of blood cells. Cambridge, Harvard University Press 1988.

25 Murre C, McCaw PS, Baltimore D: A new DNA binding and dimerization motif in immunoglobulin enhancer binding, daughterless, MyoD, and myc proteins. Cell 1989;56:777–783.

26 Nunn MF, Seeberg PH, Moscovici C, Duesberg PH: Tripartite structure of the avian erythroblastosis virus E26 transforming gene. Nature 1983;306:391–395.

27 Peters CWB, Sippel AE, Vingron M, Klempnauer KH: Drosophila and vertebrate myb proteins share two conserved regions, one of which functions as a DNA-binding domain. EMBO J 1987; 6:3085–3090.

28 Prendergast GC, Ziff EB: DNA-binding motif. Nature 1989;341:392.

29 Rauscher FJ III, Sambucetti L, Curran T, Distel RJ, Spiegelman BM: A common DNA binding site for *fos* protein complexes and transcription factor AP-1. Cell 1988; 52:471–480.

30 Rogers S, Wells R, Rechsteiner M: Amino acid sequences common to rapidly degraded proteins: The PEST hypothesis. Science 1986;234:364.

31 Sakura H, Kanei-Ishii C, Nagase T, Nakagoshi H, Gonda TJ, Ishii S: Delineation of three functional domains of the transcriptional activator encoded by the c-*myb* protooncogene. Proc Natl Acad Sci USA 1989;86:5758–5762.

32 Sap J, Munoz A, Damm K, Goldberg Y, Ghysdael J, Leutz A, Beug H, Vennström B: The c-erb-A protein is a high-affinity receptor for thyroid hormone. Nature 1986; 324:635–640.

33 Seedorf K, Krämmer G, Dürst M, Suhai S, Röwekamp WG: Human papillomavirus type 16 DNA sequence. Virology 1985;145:181–185.

34 Sommercorn J, Mulligan JA, Lozeman FJ, Krebs EG: Activation of casein kinase II in response to insulin and to epidermal growth factor. Proc Natl Acad Sci USA 1987; 84:8834.

35 Stanton LW, Schwab M, Bishop JM: Nucleotide sequence of the human N-*myc* gene. Proc Natl Acad Sci USA 1986;83:1772–1776.

36 Umesono K, Evans RM: Determinants of target gene specificity for steroid/thyroid hormone receptors. Cell 1989;57:1139–1146.

37 Van Beveren C, van Straaten F, Curran T, Müller R, Verma IM: Analysis of FBJ-MuSV provirus and c-fos (mouse) gene reveals that viral and cellular fos gene products have different carboxy termini. Cell 1983;32:1241–1255.

38 Van Ormondt H, Maat J, Dijkema R: Comparison of nucleotide sequences of the early E1a regions for subgroups A, B, and C of human adenoviruses. Gene 1980; 12:63–76.

39 Watson DK, Psallidopoulos MC, Samuel KP, Dalla-Favera R, Papas TS: Nucleotide sequence analysis of human c-myc locus, chicken homoglue and myelocytomatosis virus MC29 transforming gene reveals a highly conserved gene product. Proc Natl Acad Sci USA 1983;80:3642–3645.

40 Weston K, Bishop JM: Transcriptional activation by the v-myb oncogene and its cellular progenitor, c-myb. Cell 1989;58:85–93.

41 Battey J, Moulding C, Taub R, Murphy W, Stewart T, Potter H, Lenoir G, Leder P: The human c-myc oncogene: Structural consequences of translocation into the IgH locus in Burkitt lymphoma. Cell 1983;34:779–787.

B. Lüscher, Fred Hutchinson Cancer Research Center,
1124 Columbia Street, Seattle, WA, 98104 (USA)

Contrib Oncol, vol 39, pp 35–43 (Karger, Basel, 1990)

The *int*-1 and *int*-4 Genes in MMTV-Induced Mouse Mammary Tumors

Roel Nusse

Howard Hughes Medical Institute, Stanford University, CA, USA

Mouse mammary tumor virus (MMTV) can induce mammary tumors in susceptible mouse strains after a long latency period (4 – 12 months). The tumorinducing properties of MMTV are intrinsically related to an obligatory step in the retroviral life cycle: Insertion of proviral DNA into the host cell DNA. Integration is a mutagenic event for the host cells and one consequence may bc the activation of proto-oncogenes whose expression is normally tightly regulated [14, 15]. Additional events either or not incited by MMTV may contribute essential steps as well.

Most genes activated by MMTV, with the exception of *hst* [2], are not involved in other types of tumors and have been discovered by using MMTV DNA as a tag to clone integration domains. When multiple insertions in the same domain are found in individual tumors, there is usually an oncogene in the vicinity. By operational definition the oncogenes activated by insertion have been termed *int* genes.

This tagging strategy has now led to the identification of four such common integration domains, called *int*-1 through *int*-4. The subsequent identification of the relevant oncogene in the cloned domain has been relatives straightforward in case of *int*-1 and *int*-2, the first two genes which were discovered through this approach [5, 17]. This was facilitated by the multitude of different proviruses found near these genes in individual tumors and by their mode of insertion: proviruses were found at each end of *int*-1 or *int*-2 usually pointing away from the gene itself. This configuration hinted to the presence of a relevant gene be in between; transcripts were indeed found in those tumors with a nearby insertion and the genes were later shown to have growth regulatory properties. Strikingly, all proviral insertions mapped at any of the *int* loci leave the protein encoding domains intact, although quite a few inserts are within the transcription units. The typical orientation and the large distance of some proviruses from the *int*-1 or *int*-2 promoter indicate that the transcriptional activation of the *int* genes is mediated by enhancers in the MMTV genome, acting on the *int* promoters. The promoter of *int*-1 has been mapped and is indeed similarly active in tumors as in cells where the genes are naturally expressed, except for rare cases with proviral insertions within the promoter. The typical orientation of MMTV proviruses near *int*-1 and *int*-2 [5, 16] is explained by the relative inefficiency of enhancers to work on a second promoter encountered *in cis*.

The int-1 Gene

In the C3H mouse strain, 70 – 80 % of the MMTV induced mammary tumors contain an MMTV provirus integration activating the *int*-1 gene [16, 17]. In these tumors a 2.6 kb mRNA is found, which is absent in normal mammary tissue. The *int*-1 gene is unusually highly conserved in evolution, having a virtually identical human homolog and easily recognizable amphibian and insect counterparts. *Int*-1 encodes a protein with many cysteine residues and a signal peptide but without a transmembrane domain. These are properties of secretory proteins, and *int*-1 protein species, if overexpressed in various cell lines, are indeed seen to enter the secretory pathway, and contains carbohydrate structures at several N-linked glycosylation sites [2, 18, 19]. *Int*-1 has never been detected in culture medium. Recently is has been shown that *int*-1 overproduction in CHO cells leads to small amounts of extracellular protein which has undergone more extensive glycosylations and may bind to the cell surface or to the extracellular matrix possibly explaining its absence in free form in tissue culture medium [18].

A problem in studying mouse *int*-1 protein is its weak antigenicity. A solution to this problem has been found in *Drosophila*, where *int*-1 is identical to the segment polarity gene *wingless*. The mouse and *Drosophila* *int*-1 proteins are identical in 54 % of their amino acids, but the *Drosophila* gene has an insert encoding an additional 85 amino acids. Antibodies raised to the D*int*-1-*wingless* protein are able to detect the protein in whole mount embryos and in individual cells, and it is probably the insert that has provided the highly antigenic determinant. Secretion of the *wingless* protein has been observed in the electron microscope, where the protein is seen in small membrane bound vesicles, in multivesicular bodies and in the intercellular space [28]. Traveling of the protein is suggested by an experiment employing double staining of wildtype embryos with both *wingless* and *engrailed* antibodies. The *engrailed* protein is located in the nucleus of cells immediately posterior to the *wingless* cells. The multivesicular bodies containing the wingless protein are occasionally found in engrailed positive cells, suggesting that the wingless protein behaves as a paracrine signal [28].

All in all, it seems that *int*-1 is indeed secreted like any other secretory molecule. When the gene is overexpressed however, proper folding of the protein may not occur, resulting in retention as an aggregate in the ER. This aggregation has frustrated many attempts to purify biologically active *int*-1 protein from mammalian or insect cells.

Experimental evidence ofr an *int*-1 receptor has not been obtained, but given the secretion of the protein, we can expect that the *int*-1 receptor will behave like other growth factor receptors: binding its ligand on the cell surface followed by internalization.

int-1 expression patterns and role in embryogenesis

In adult mice, *int*-1 is not expressed in any tissue, except for the mature testis [8, 25]. Expression is localized in post-meiotic, round spermatids, but the biological role of this expression in unclear. In mouse embryos, *int*-1 is expressed between day 8 and day 14, specifically in the developing nervous system [30]. Areas in the neural plate, the anterior head folds, the folding neural tube and the spinal cord show a highly localized expression of *int*-1. During folding of the neural tube, expression moves from anterior to posterior. Also in *Xenopus* embryos, *int*-1 expression is associated with neural development [13]. It has been suggested that the gene is involved in positional signaling in the developing neural system, providing information specifying the midline axis. In line with this view are the dramatic effects on the developing *Xenopus* embryos when *int*-1 RNA is injected into fertilized eggs: a bifurcating anterior neural tube and expansion of the posterior neural plate. In addition the underlying axial mesoderm is duplicated, suggesting dual formation of the whole embryonic axis perhaps as a result of interference with the so-called organizer [11].

Most tested embryonal carcinoma cell lines do not express *int*-1, except for the P19 cells when induced by retinoic acid to differentiate into the neural pathway [24].

Developmental mutations at int-1 in Drosophila

When the *Drosophila* homolog of *int*-1 was cloned, it turned out to be identical to the segment polarity gene *wingless* [1, 22]. From clonal analysis of *wingless* cells, it appeared that the phenotype is non-autonomous in mosaics, which suggests that the protein has a role in intercellular signaling. Various alleles of *wingless* are known. A viable allele, which gave the gene its name, leads to a homeotic transformation of the wing into a notum. Embryonic lethal alleles cause more severe effects, such as the absence of segment boundaries and an inverted polarity of the posterior zone of each segment [1]. Expression of *wingless* has been localized both with *in situ* RNA hybridization and with immunostaining. The gene is expressed in regions which are aberrantly developed in *wingless* mutants: different regions of the head, the hindgut/anal region and in 15 stripes in the trunk region. After gastrulation, expression is seen in each segment, in a few cells just anterior to the parasegment boundary [1, 28].

The genetics of *Drosophila* segmentation may offer an alternative approach to find an *int*-1 receptor: the phenotype of a *wingless* receptor mutant may be similar to *wingless* itself, and at least eight genes with such a phenotype have been characterized. Some of those mutants behave in a cell autonomous way, which would also be expected of a receptor gene. As many of these genes are now being cloned (reviewed in [7]), more information will soon become available. Further genetic and biochemical analysis of *wingless* in the process of segmentation and in outgrowth of imaginal discs will undoubtedly help to elucidate the signal transduction pathway in which the gene is involved, with obvious ramifications to the mechanism of action of *int*-1 in the mouse. Several circuits of such interactions have been proposed, including expression of the nuclear protein *engrailed* in target cells [6], transcriptional repression of *wingless* by the pair-rule genes *even-skipped* and *fushi-tarazu* and inhibition of *wingless* action by expression of the membrane protein *patched* [12].

Assays for int-1 activity

There are now several biological assays based on *int*-1 activity. The most dramatic effects of the gene are seen *in vivo*, in intact animals. The effects of ectopic expression of *int*-1 RNA in Xenopus embryos have already been mentioned. In the mouse, a transgene consisting of *int*-1 with an MMTV LTR inserted upstream and in the opposite orientation as the gene, causes massive proliferation of mammary epithelial cells, resulting in hyperplastic glands [26]. Those mice are not able to nurse their offspring. After a period of latency, mammary tumors emerge in astochastic pattern, presumably by somatic mutations. The hyperplasia in *int*-1 transgenic mice also occurs in males, which is a unique aspect of *int*-1; male mice carrying other oncogenes linked to the MMTV LTR are usually normal.

Transgenic flies with the *wingless* gene under a heat shock promoter display interesting phenotypes during embryogenesis. The most extreme phenotype is a naked cuticle, which is, not unexpectedly, the opposite of the *wingless* phenotype (J. Noordermeer, P. Lawrence and R. Nusse, unpublished).

The *in vitro* effects of *int*-1 are less spectacular. By retroviral or direct gene transfer, two cell lines from mammary origin can be morphologically transformed. these cells, called C57MG and RAC, normally have a cuboidal phenotype, grow to a low density and are not tumorigenic. Upon uptake and overexpression of *int*-1 constructs, the cells become elongated, form foci, and in case of the RAC cells, grow as tumors in suitable recipient mice [3, 23]. These effects are not seen when fibroblastic lines are used, and hint to a cell type specificity of *int*-1 transforming ability. A problem with these assays is that the transformed cells are quite unlike mamary tumor cells with activated *int*-1; they lack most markers of mammary cells and the tumors growing out of the transfected RAC cells are pathologically different from primary mouse mammary tumors. The full spectrum of *int*-1 activity may thus not be completely represented by these in vitro transformed cells.

int-1 related genes: int-4 and irp

int-4 gene, also identified by provirus tagging methods, is rather infrequently activated by MMTV, only in five individual tumors all from GR mice. The size of the transcriptional unit, which appears to cover more than 50 Kb, has complicated its structural analysis. Sequence analysis has shown the *int*-4 encoded protein to show extensive homology with *int*-1; particularly striking is the conservation of all cysteine residues (H. Roelink and R. Nusse, unpublished). *int*-4 is normally expressed in mouse embryos as a 3.8 kb mRNA, probably in the developing brain, and in differentiating P19 embryonal carcinoma cells. The pattern of expression in rather similar to *int*-1.

The *irp* gene was encountered by Wrainwright et al. [29] who were in search for a gene predisposing to cystic fibrosis (CF) on human chromosome 7 by a chromosome walk. *Irp* is not the CF gene, but shows 38% identity with *int*-1 with all cysteines conserved, hence the name *int*-1 related protein.

In view of the homology with *int*-1, we have recently examined whether m-*irp* can also behave as an oncogene in mouse mammary tumors. No cases of tumors with MMTV insertions near the gene were found, but two tumors appeared to have amplified copies of *irp*. In those tumors, which were negative for *int*-1 activation, considerable overexpression of *irp* was detected, suggesting that amplification of *irp* had been instrumental in tumorgenesis.

Conclusion

In embryogenesis the *int* genes may function in pattern formation by encoding secreted proteins with a short range of action, influencing the fate of surrounding cells or tissues.

In resuming all what is known on the *int* genes, one wonders why these virally induced mouse mammary tumors arise by activation of developmental genes, and hardly or not by activation of a more clasical oncogene. In other words, why is *myc* or c-*erb*B-2 never activated, whereas these and many other oncogenes are capable of inducing mouse mammary tumors, if present as a transgene? Apparently, the mouse mammary gland is extremely sensitive to the inadvertent expression of an *int* gene. Obviously, the mamary cells mus have receptors for the *int* genes, but is is unlikely that they are the only cells equipped with such receptors, nor can we assume that mammary cells would not have receptors for other oncogene products.

It may be that developmental genes are potent mammary oncogenes because the tumors arise in a developing organ: only in mammary glands cycling through multiple rounds of pregnancy. In this aspect, the mammary gland is unique among the adult organs, which may explain the unique association of abnormal mammary growth with ectopic activation of developmental genes. The major mitogenic stimulus in tumorigenesis comes then from pregnancy hormones [9], and aberrant growth may result from activation of genes controling normal growth at an abnormal point in life.

Combinatorial activity of the *int* genes with other factors could explain their seemingly contrasting functions in normal development and in mammary tumorigenesis. During development, the *int* genes are expressed in areas with no or a low rate of proliferation and then they probably only act as morphogens, inducing differentiation in embryonic tissue. Upon inadvertent activation by MMTV in mammary tissue, they may, in conjunction with other factors, act as strong mitogens. The combined activation of *int*-1 and *int*-2 in some mammary tumors is therefore of particular interest. The end result of the activity of many growth factors depends on the context in which these factors are present.

It is anticipated that new insight into the mechanism of action of the *int* genes will be generated by inactivating the genes in the mouse germ line and examining the phenotype of the resulting mutant mice. The possibility to manipulate embryonic stem cells *in vitro* to introduce mutations at will by homologous recombination has been explored for both *int*-1 and *int*-2. For *int*-2, such mutations have been obtained at a relatively high frequency [10], whereas very few homologous recombinants at *int*-1 were generated [4]. This contrast may be due to differences in expression levels of the genes in embryonic stem cells, since the selection procedures used depend in part on the transcirptional capacity of the target locus. To date however, no mice bearing a germ line mutation at one of the *int* loci have been generated. Once obtained, such animals will be invaluable in examining the tasks of these intriguing genes in the developing animal, and, by extrapolation, in the process of mammary tumorigenesis.

References

1   Baker NE: Molecular cloning of sequences from wingless, a segment polarity gene in Drosophila: the spatial distribution of a transcript in embryos. EMBO J 1987;6:1765-1773.

2   Brown AMC, Papkoff J, Fung YKT, Shacklefort GM, Varmus HE: Identification of protein products encoded by the proto-oncogene int-1. Mol Cell Biol 1987;7:3971-3977.

3   Brown AMC, Wildin RS, Prendergast TJ, Varmus HE: A retrovirus vector expressing the putative mammary oncogene int-1 causes partial transformation of a mammary epithelial cell line. Cell 1986;46:1001-1009.

4   Capecchi MR: The new mouse genetics: Altering the genome by gene targeting. Trends Genet 1989;5:70-76.

5   Dickson C, Smith R, Brookes S, Peters G: Tumorigenesis by mouse mammary tumor virus: Proviral activation of a cellular gene in the common integration region int-2. Cell 1984;37:529-536.

6   DiNardo S, Sher E, Heemskerk-Jongens J, Kassis JA, O'Farrell PH: Two-tiered regu-
    lation of spatially patterned engrailed gene expression during Drosophila embryo-
    genesis. Nature 1988;332:604–609.

7   Ingham PW: The molecular genetics of embryonic pattern formation in Drosophila.
    Nature 1988;335:25–34.

8   Jakobovits A, Shackleford GM, Varmus HE, Martin GR: Two proto-oncogenes
    implicated in mammary carcinogenesis, int-1 and int-2, are independently regulated
    during mouse development. Proc Natl Acad Sci USA 1986;83:7806–7810.

9   Kratochwil K: The importance of epithelial stromal interaction in mammary gland
    development, in Rich MA, Hager JC, Taylor-Papadimitrion J (eds): Breast Cancer:
    Origins, detection, and treatment. Boston, Martinus Nijhoff, 1985, pp 1–12.

10 Mansour SL, Thomas KR, Capecchi MR: Disruption of the proto-oncogene int-2 in
    mouse embryo-derived stem cells: A general strategy for targeting mutations to non-
    selectable genes. Nature 1988;336:348–352.

11 McMahon AP, Moon RT: Ectopic expression of the proto-oncogene int-1 in Xeno-
    pus embryos leads to duplication of the embryonic axis. Cell 1989;58:1075–1084.

12 Nakano Y, Guerrero I, Hildalgo A, Taylor A, Whittle JRS, Ingham PW: The Droso-
    phila segment polarity gene patched encodes a protein with multiple potential mem-
    brane spanning regions. Nature 1989;341:508–513.

13 Noordermeer J, Meijlink F, Verrijzer P, Rijsewijk F, Destree O: Isolation of the
    Xenopus homolog of int-1/wingless and expression during neurula stages of early
    development. Nucl Acids Res 1989;17:11–18.

14 Nusse R: The activation of cellular oncogenes by retroviral insertion. Trends Genet
    1986;2:244–247.

15 Nusse R: The int genes in mammary tumorigenesis and in normal development.
    Trends Genet 1988;4:291–295.

16 Nusse R, Van Ooyen A, Cox D, Fung YKT, Varmus HE: Mode of proviral activation
    of a putative mammary oncogene (int-1) on mouse chromosome 15. Nature 1984;
    307:131–136.

17 Nusse R, Varmus HE: Many tumors induced by the mouse mammary tumor virus
    contain a provirus integrated in the same region of the host genome. Cell 1982;
    31:99–109.

18 Papkoff, J: Inducible overexpression and secretion of int-1 protein. Mol Cell Biol
    1989;8:3377–3384.

19 Papkoff J, Brown AMC, Varmus HE: The int-1 proto-oncogene products are glyco-
    proteins that appear to enter the secretory pathway. Mol Cell Biol 1987;7:3978–3984.

20 Peters G, Brookes S, Smith R, Dickson C: Tumorigenesis by mouse mammary tumor
    virus: Evidence for a common region for provirus integration in mammary tumors.
    Cell 1983;33:369–377.

21 Peters G, Brookes S, Smith R, Placzek M, Dickson C: The mouse homolog of the hst/
    k-FGF gene is adjacent to int-2 and activated by proviral insertion in some virally
    induced mammary tumors. Proc Natl Acad Sci USA, 1989; in press.

22 Rijsewijk F, Schuermann M, Wagenaar E, Parren P, Weigel D, Nusse R: The Droso-
    phila homolgue of the mammary oncogene int-1 is identical to the segment polarity
    gene wingless. Cell 1987;50:649–657.

23 Rijsewijk F, Van Deemter L, Wagenaar E, Sonnenberg A, Nusse R: Transfection of the int-1 mammary oncogene in cuboidal RAC mammary cell line results in morphological transformation and tumorigenicity. EMBO J 1987;6:127–131.

24 Schuuring E, van Deemter E, Roelink H, Nusse R: Expression of the int-1 proto-oncogene during differentiation of P19 embryonal carcinoma cells. Mol Cell Biol 1989;9:1357–1361.

25 Shackleford GM, Varmus HE: Expression of the proto-oncogene int-1 is restricted to postmeiotic male germ cells and the neural tube of mid-gestational embryos. Cell 1987;50:89–95.

26 Tsukamoto AS, Grosschedl R, Guzman RC, Parslow T, Varmus HE: Expression of the int-1 gene in transgenic mice is associated with mammary gland hyperplasia and adenocarcinomas in male and female mice. Cell 1988;55:619–625.

27 Van Ooyen A, Nusse R: Structure and nucleotide sequence of the putative mammary oncogene int-1: Proviral insertions leave the protein-encoding domain intact. Cell 1984;39:233–240.

28 Van den Heuvel M, Nusse R, Johnston P, Lawrence P: Distribution of the wingless protein in Drosophila embryos: a protein involved in cell-cell interactions. Cell 1989; in press.

29 Wainwright BJ, Scambler PJ, Stanier P, Watson EK, Bell G, Wicking C, Estivill X, Courtney M, Boue A, Pedersen PS, Williamson R, Farrall M: Isolation of a human gene with protein sequence similarity to human and murine int-1 and the Drosophila segment polarity mutant wingless. EMBO J 1988;7:1743–1748.

30 Wilkinson DG, Bailes JA, McMahon AP: Expression of the proto-oncogene int-1 is restricted to specific neural cells in the developing mouse embryo. Cell 1987; 50:79–88.

Roel Nusse, Howard Hughes Medical Institute, Beckman Center B 202, Stanford University Medical Center, Stanford, CA 94305-5428, USA

Contrib Oncol, vol 39, pp 44–51 (Karger, Basel, 1990)

RAS Oncogenes as Tools to Study Tumor Development

J. L. Bos

Department of Molecular Carcinogenesis, Sylvius Laboratories, Leiden, the Netherlands

Mutated RAS Genes in Human Tumors

The RAS gene family consists of three members, the HRAS, the KRAS, and the NRAS gene. They are identified as activated oncogenes by their ability to transform NIH/3T3 cells. The transforming property is due to point mutations which are located in codons 12, 13 and 61 [1].

We have analyzed tumor DNAs for the presence of a mutated RAS gene by selective hybridization of PCR-amplified material with synthetic oligonucleotides [3]. A summary of our results as presented in table 1 allow us to make the following conclusions:

1. Mutated RAS genes are found in a variety of malignancies, both in solid tumors and in leukemias. However, in a large number of tumor types, no RAS gene mutation has been found or they occur only sporadically, indicating that there is a certain specificity in the type of malignancies where RAS gene mutations occur. This specificity is shown most strikingly in lung tumors, where we find RAS gene mutations in 30 % of the adenocarcinomas, but not in squamous cell carcinomas or in large cell carcinomas. All three tumor types, however, may originate from a similar cell type, the bronchiolog-alviolar epithelial cell. The reason for this difference in specificity is still unclear.

2. There is some specificity in the type of RAS gene mutated. In most solid tumors KRAS is the predominantly activated gene, whereas in hematopoietic malignancies NRAS is most frequently activated. The specificity in RAS gene mutations is most prominent in pancreatic tumors, where only KRAS mutations have been observed thus far. HRAS gene mutations are found infrequently in human tumors.

Table 1. Incidence of RAS gene mutations in human tumors

Tumor type*	incidence**	RAS***
Breast	0	
Ovary	0	
Cervix	0	
Esophageal	0	
Glioblastoma	0	
Lung		
Epidermoid carcinoma	0	
Large cell carcinoma	0	
Adenocarcinoma	30	KRAS
Colon		
Adenoma	50	KRAS
Adenocarcinoma	50	KRAS
Pancreas	85	KRAS
Seminoma	40	N-, KRAS
Melanoma	20	KRAS
Myeloid		
MDS	30	NRAS
AML	30	NRAS
CML	0	
Lymphoid		
ALL	10	NRAS
CLL	0	
NHL	0	

For references, see Bos, 1989.
  *Indicated are results from our laboratory and collaborators only.
 **Percentage of tumors harboring a mutant RAS gene.
***RAS gene preferentially activated.

3. Mutated RAS genes are not restricted to malignant tumors. They occur in premalignant lesions as well, for instance, in colon adenomas and in myelodysplastic syndrome or preleukemia.

4. In those tumor types where a RAS gene mutation has been detected, the incidence varies greatly. The highest incidence, thus far, is found in adenocarcinomas of the pancreas, but mostly incidences between 20 and 50% are observed. This raises the question whether there is a difference between tumors that have RAS mutations and those that do not. Extensive analysis of clinical and histo-pathological features of mutated RAS positive and mutated RAS negative tumors does not reveal clear differences, how-

ever. This implies that there is no absolute requirement for RAS activation during the development of a tumor and that other genetic events can occur which have a more or less similar effect in tumor development as RAS gene mutations. Moreover, tumor development is a multistep process and the ultimate tumor is the result of the accumulation of a variety of genetic changes. It is therefore conceivable that a mutated RAS gene does not provide a unique feature to a tumor.

Several tumor types have been analyzed extensively with respect to the presence of mutated RAS genes. This has provided some insight in the heterogeneity of tumors, the timing of the mutational event and the possible involvement of chemical mutagens in the induction of the mutation. I will present some examples.

Myelodysplastic syndrome and acute myeloid leukemia

Myeloid leukemia can be divided into three main groups of diseases, myelodysplastic syndrome (MDS) or preleukemia, acute myeloid leukemia (AML) and chronic myeloid leukemia (CML). MDS is a heterogeneous group of disorders characterized by abnormally low counts of one or more of the blood lineages and bone marrow abnormalities. It may progress into AML in one-third of the cases. Most likely, the initiating event in this disease affects an early stem cell and the subsequent progression is marked by the accumulation of chromosome abnormalities and the gradual increase of blast cells. Arbitrarily, patients with more than 30 % immature blast cells in their bone marrow are diagnosed as having AML. We [4, 9] and others [2, 5, 7] have found that 30 % of the MDS and AML patients have a mutated RAS gene in their (pre) leukemic cells.

From studies in which multiple samples have been analyzed from the same patient we have obtained information at which stage of the disease the mutational event can occur [9] (fig. 1). In one group of patients the mutation is present early in the course of the disease and can be detected in both the affected and the unaffected blood cell lineages, such as the peripheral lymphocytes, suggesting that the mutational event has occurred in a multipotent stem cell, the precursor for all lineages. During complete clinical remission, cells with a mutated RAS gene are still present and may comprise a major fraction of the bone marrow cells. In a subsequent relapse the mutation is still present in the leukemic cell clone. In a second group of patients the mutation is not present in the initial phase of the disease, but

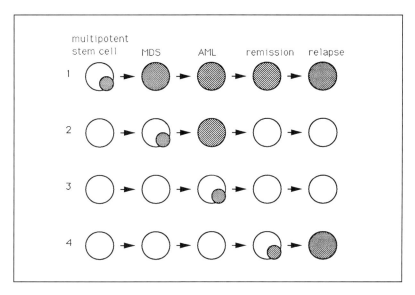

Fig. 1. Schematic representation of the various stages of myeloid leukemia with the occurrance of RAS gene mutations. (The presence of a mutated RAS gene is indicated by the gray circles). 1: The RAS gene mutation occurs in a multipotent stem cell and in most cases resists chemotherapy. 2 and 3: The RAS gene mutation occurs in a preleukemic cell (2) or in an already leukemic cell (3), resulting in the development of a new, more malignant cell clone. This cell clone is mostly destroyed during treatment. 4: The RAS gene mutation occurs during the remission phase of the disease and is responsible for the subsequent relapse.

occurs during the course of the disease. Initially, a mutated RAS gene is only detected in a subfraction of the bone marrow cells, but gradually the fraction of RAS containing cells increases, more or less concomitant with the increase in immature blast cells. Apparently in these patients the mutated RAS gene is present in a newly evolving leukemic cell clone, which is the major cell clone during the acute phase of the disease. At clinical remission, no mutated RAS genes can be detected in the bone marrow and also in a subsequent relapse no mutated RAS genes are present. This indicates that during treatment the cell clone harboring the mutated RAS gene is killed. Although these two groups comprise the majority of the MDS patients with a mutated RAS gene, there are variations on this theme. For instance, in some patients the mutated RAS gene has only been found in the relapse and not in the initial leukemia and in some patients two different RAS gene mutations have been found, probably in two different cell clones.

From these results we conclude that the mutational event in MDS/AML may be an early or even initial event as well as an event which may occur during the progression of the disease. Furthermore we can conclude that mutant RAS containing cell clones in patients with a mutation in a multipotent stem cell appears to be more resistant to chemotherapy than cell clones where the mutations had occured later in the course of the disease.

Melanomas

Melanomas are highly malignant tumor which metastasize very rapidly. The incidence of RAS mutations is approximately 20 %. The analysis of these tumors for the presence of mutated RAS genes resulted in a striking observation with respect to heterogeneity in the tumor [8]. We found in two tumors two different mutated RAS alleles, whereas in the metastasis of the same tumors only one of the mutated alleles was present. In one case both the mutated alleles were identified in different metastasis. This implies that the primary tumor consists of two different cell clones, each with a mutated RAS gene and each with metastatic potential. A model to explain the generation of the two cell clones is presented in figure 2.

We hypothesize that one of the latest events in the formation of the primary tumor is a genetic lesion in the RAS gene. During replication of this lesion a mutation in the strand opposite of the lesion occurs and, thus, one of the daughter cells contains a mutation. When the lesion persists, in the next round of replication another mutation can occur opposite the lesion. This will result in two cell clones which are phenotypically similar, but different in the RAS gene mutation. Alternatively, the two cell clones are independent tumors or independent malignant subclones of a premalignant lesion.

An indication that specific DNA lesions are responsible for the induction of the RAS gene mutation comes from the observation that all primary melanomas in which we have found a RAS gene mutation are located at sites continuously exposed to sunlight (see table 2), indicating that UV-light (which generates pyrimidine dimers) may be the etiological agent for the induction of RAS mutations.

Seminomas

Seminomas are germline tumors of the testis. We have found that in 40 % of the tumors a mutated RAS gene can be detected, but in most cases

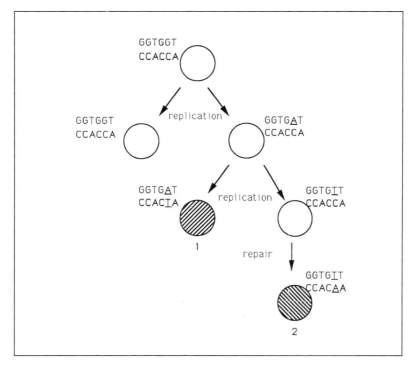

Fig. 2. Model for the formation of two different cell clones with respect to mutated RAS alleles in primary melanomas. Due to DNA damage, for instance cytidine dimerization, a mispairing occurs opposite the lesion, resulting in a cell clone with a RAS gene mutation (1) When the lesion persists a second cell line can be generated with a different RAS gene mutation (2).

the mutation was present in only a subfraction of the cells [6]. To exclude that infiltrating lymphocytes and normal stromal cells are the cause of this observation, we separated the aneuploid nuclei of the tumor cells from the diploid nuclei of the non-tumor cells by flow sorting. Even after this purification of tumor cell nuclei, the mutation was found to be present in a subfraction of the cells only. In some tumors, we could detect areas which do not contain mutant RAS genes, whereas in other areas a mutated RAS gene is clearly present. However, both the histopathology and the DNA index of the different areas of such a tumor are identical. This indicates that the different areas represent the same primary tumor. Several explanations can be put forward to explain these results (see fig. 3): First, the RAS mutation has occurred late in the course of tumor formation and the cell clone con-

Table 2. Relation between the site of the primary melanoma with respect to sunlight exposure and the presence of RAS gene mutations

Sunlight exposure of site of primary tumor	Number of tumors tested	Tumors with mutated RAS gene
Continuous	10	7
Intermittent	16	0
Rare	5	0
Unknown	6	0

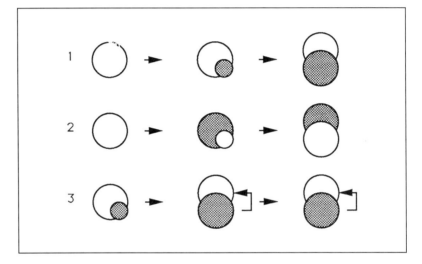

Fig. 3. Three possible explanations for the genetic heterogeneity with respect to RAS gene mutations in seminomas. Indicated are cell clones with (gray) and without (white) mutant RAS genes. 1: RAS gene mutations are present in a new sublone of the tumor and provides this clone which a slight growth advantage, but has not yet repopulated the whole tumor mass. 2: RAS gene mutations occur during the early stages of tumor development, but are lost during progression. 3: RAS gene mutations are present in a subclone of the tumor and result in the secretion of growth factors which can also stimulate the non-RAS containing tumor cells in a paracrine fashion.

taining the RAS mutation represents a new cell clone with some growth advantage. The mutational event is not sufficient to give the new cell clone a different morphology, however. A second possibility is that initially a tumor cell harbored the mutated RAS gene, but that it is gradually lost during the development of the tumor. In this case the mutated RAS gene has played a role in the initial stages of the disease only. A final explanation could be that mutated RAS genes occurred at a relatively late stage of tumor development and resulted in a cell clone which produced a growth factor giving growth advantage to both the mutant RAS-containing cells and the cells that did not contain a mutated RAS gene. This would result in a mixed population of cells with respect to the presence of mutated RAS genes.

From the above examples it is clear that the analysis of RAS point mutations in human tumors may not yet provide valuable information with respect to clinical applications, but does provide new insights in the mechanism of tumor formation.

Acknowledgement

This work was supported by the Dutch Cancer Foundation. I thank Frank McCormick for reading the manuscript.

References

1   Barbacid M: *Ras* genes. Ann Rev. Biochem 1987;56:776–827.
2   Bartam CR, Ludwig WD, Hiddeman W, Lyons J, Buschle M, Ritter J, Harbot J, Fröhlich A, Janssen JWG: Acute myeloid leukemia: analysis of *ras* gene mutations and clonality defined by polymorphic X-linked loci. Leukemia 1989;3:247–256.
3   Bos JL: Ras oncogenes in human cancer: A review. Cancer Res 1989;49:4682–4689.
4   Bos JL, Verlaan-de Vries M, Van der Eb AJ, Janssen JWG, Delwel R, Löwenberg B, Colly LP: Mutations in N-*ras* predominate in acute myeloid leukemia. Blood 1987; 69:1237–1241.
5   Farr CJ, Saiki RK, Erlich HA, McCormick F, Marshall CJ: Analysis of *ras* gene mutations in acute myeloid leukemia using the polymerase chain reaction and oligonucleotide probes. Proc Natl Acad Sci USA 1988;85:1629–1633.
6   Mulder MP, Keijzer W, Verkerk A, Boot AJM, Prins MEF, Splinter TAW, Bos JL: Activated ras genes in human seminoma: evidence for tumor heterogeneity. Oncogene 1989;4:1345–1351.
7   Padua RA, Carter G, Hughes D, Gow J, Farr C, Orcier D, McCormick F, Jacobs A: *Ras* mutations in myelodysplasia detected by amplification, oligonucleotide hybridization, and transformation. Leukemia 1988;2:503–510.
8   Van't Veer LJ, Burgering BMT, Versteeg R, Boot AJM, Ruiter DJ, Osanto S, Schrier PI, Bos JL: N-*ras* mutations in human cutaneous melanoma correlated with sun exposure. Mol Cell Biol 1989;9:3114–3116.
9   Yunis JJ, Boot AJM, Mayer MG, Bos JL: Mechanism of *ras* mutation in myelodysplastic syndrome. Oncogene 1989;4:609–614.

J.L. Bos, Department of Molecular Carcinogenesis, Sylvius Laboratories, Wassenaarseweg 72, NL-2333 AL Leiden (The Netherlands)

Contrib Oncol, vol 39, pp 52–59 (Karger, Basel, 1990)

Expression of Epstein-Barr Virus Latent Genes and Evidence for Integration of Viral DNA into the Host Genome in Burkitt's Lymphoma Cells

U. Zimber-Strobl[a, b], *K. O. Suentzenich,*[a, b] *G. Laux*[b], *M. Cordier*[c],
A. Calender[c], *M. Billaud*[c], *G. M. Lenoir*[c], *G. W. Bornkamm*[a, b]

[a] Abtl. Virologie, Inst. f. Med. Mikrobiologie, Universtität Freiburg, FRG
[b] Inst. f. Klin. Molekularbiologie u. Tumorgenetik, Hämatologikum der GSF, München, FRG
[c] International Agency for Research on Cancer, Lyon, France

Burkitt's lymphoma is a human B cell malignancy with particular high incidence in tropical Africa. It occurs with 20 to 50 fold lower incidence in all other parts of the world. The tumor is characterized by chromosomal translocations involving the c-myc locus on chromosome 8 and one of the immunoglobulin heavy or light chain genes [2]. In addition, almost all african and about 15 % of the non-african tumors carry Epstein-Barr virus (EBV) DNA and express at least one viral antigen, the nuclear antigen EBNA1. The association of EBV with Burkitt's lymphoma suggests that EBV is important, although not compulsory in the development of the disease, providing one factor in the multistep development of cancer [7]. With regard to the cooperativity of oncogenes it is important to know which viral gene functions, if any, are involved in the development of Burkitt's lymphoma.

EBNA2 induces expression of B cell activation markers

Since EBV is capable of inducing proliferation in normal human B cells, it was suggestive to assume that viral gene functions involved in induction of lymphoproliferation in normal cells would also be associated with the development of Burkitt's lymphoma. In EBV transformed cells at least 9 viral proteins are expressed. Of these, 6 are located in the nucleus

(EBNA1, 2, 3A, 3B, 3C, LP) and 3 in the membrane (LMP, TP1, TP2) (fig. 1). We focussed our attention initially on viral genes deleted in the non-transforming EBV strain P3HR-1. This work resulted in the mapping of the deletion in P3HR-1 virus at the boundary of the large internal repeats to the long unique region of the virus genome and in the identification of EBNA2 as a gene encoded by the deleted region [1, 10]. EBNA2 plays a crucial role in changing the phenotype and the pattern of gene expression of EBV infected cells as shown by Calender et al. [3]. The authors compared the phenotype of EBV negative Burkitt's lymphoma cells with that of cells infected with a transformation-defective virus carrying the EBNA2 deletion (P3HR-1), and of cells infected with a transformation-competent, EBNA2 expressing virus (B95–8). B95–8 virus convertants, in contrast to EBV negative Burkitt's lymphoma cells and P3HR-1 virus converted cells, express high levels of B cell activation markers such as the receptor for the

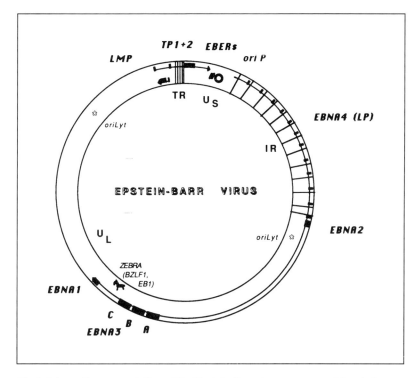

Fig. 1. Schematic representation of the Epstein-Barr virus genome and the viral genes expressed in growth-transformed cells. The viral genome is circularized via the terminal repetitions.

complement component C3d (CD21) and the low affinity FcE receptor CD23. These molecules have been implicated in the control of B cell proliferation. To demonstrate the role of EBNA2 in the induction of CD 21 and CD23, we have stably introduced the EBNA2 gene on an episomal vector into P3HR-1 virus converted BL41 cells [4]. All EBNA2 expressing cell clones showed significantly higher levels of CD21 and CD23 transcripts and expressed higher levels of the gene products either on the cell surface (CD21) or shed into the medium (CD23) suggesting that EBNA2 is transactivating the genes coding for CD21 and CD23 (table 1).

EBNA2 is not Expressed in EBV positive Burkitt's Lymphoma Cells in vivo

The great potential of EBNA2 to change the pattern of gene expression and to alter the phenotype of human B lymphocytes raises a paradox regarding the role of EBV in the development of Burkitt's lymphoma. On one hand, looking at tumor biopsies, EBV positive and EBV negative Burkitt's lymphomas are indistinguishable with regard to cell morphology and phenotype. On the other hand, wild type EBV alters the cell morphology, the cell surface phenotype and the growth pattern in a dramatic fashion,

Table 1. Expression of viral antigens and B cell activation markers in EBV converted cell lines

	BL 41	BL41-P3	BL41-B95	BL41-P3 EBNA2 transfected
EBNA1	−	+	+	+
EBNA2	−	−	+	(+)
LMP	−	−	+	−
CD21 (RNA)	low	low	high	increased
CD21 (surface)	low	low	high	increased
CD23 (surface)	low	low	high	increased
CD23 (surface)	low	low	high	low
CD23 (soluble)	low	low	high	increased
T cell cytotoxicity	−	−	+	n. d.

(+) indicates low expression

when studied in vitro. This apparent paradox was recently resolved by Rickinson and coworkers, who could show that cells obtained from biopsies differ significantly in morphology, phenotype, growth pattern and viral gene expression from those of Burkitt's lymphoma cells established as cell lines in tissue culture [12]. Cells from biopsies do not express EBNA2 and the latent membrane protein (LMP), have the phenotype CD10$^+$, CDw77$^+$, CD21$^-$, Cd23$^-$, CD30$^-$, and grow in single cell suspension. However, most EBV positive cell lines in culture express EBNA2 and LMP as well as activation markers such as CD21, CD23 and CD30, and grow in large clumps [13, 14]. Only a minority of EBV positive Burkitt's lymphomas have maintained their original phenotype and growth pattern even after long term culture in vitro. Such lines may be taken as a model reflecting the pattern of viral gene expression in the in vivo situation. The lack of expression of EBNA2 and LMP in Burkitt's lymphoma biopsies may also explain the missing T cell response against EBV carrying Burkitt's lymphoma cells *in vivo*, since EBNA2 and EBNA2-induced viral and cellular proteins are involved in T cell defense mechanisms, either by serving as targets for cytotoxic T cells or by mediating cell-ccll interaction [9, 11].

Expression of the EBV terminal protein gene is dependent on EBNA2

The finding that ENBA2 is not expressed in EBV positive Burkitt's lymphoma cells in vivo has turned the attention to other viral genes. One of these genes, potentially involved in tumor development is the one coding for the terminal proteins TP1 and TP2. The exons of this gene are located at both ends of the linear viral genome and generate a functional transcription unit only if the viral DNA is circularized [6, 15]. To study expression of the terminal protein gene in Burkitt's lymphoma cells we have generated an S1 probe from a TP1 cDNA spanning the junction between exon 1 and exon 2. This probe protects a fragment of 327 b corresponding to the TP1 message and a fragment of 150 b corresponding to TP2 mRNA. Analysis of a large panel of Burkitt's lymphoma cell lines for expression of the terminal protein gene revealed a number of interesting findings:

1. TP expression was highly variable from no or very low expression in some Burkitt's lymphoma lines to high expression in most other lines.

2. TP1 RNA was the major TP RNA species whereas TP2 RNA could only be detected in a minority of cell lines.

3. The attempt to correlate TP expression with the phenotype of Burkitt's lymphoma cell lines revealed a strong correlation between TP and EBNA2 expression. EBNA2 negative cell lines, which had maintained the in vivo phenotype of Burkitt's lymphoma cells, expressed no or very little amounts of TP, whereas EBNA2 positive cell lines were invariably positive for TP expression.

The correlation between EBNA2 and TP expression was further strengthened by studying TP expression in P3HR-1 and B95-8 virus converted EBV negative Burkitt's lymphoma lines. All P3HR-1 virus convertants were negative for TP expression and all B95-8 virus convertants positive. Furthermore, introduction of the EBNA2 gene into P3HR-1 virus converted BL41 cells induced TP expression. Constructs containing either the TP1 or TP2 promoter in front of the chloramphenicolacetyltransferase (CAT) gene were inactive in EBV negative and P3HR-1 virus-converted cells, and were highly active in B95-8 virus convertants. This suggests that EBNA2 is transactivating the TP1 as well as the TP2 promoter.

These findings illustrate the importance of EBNA2 as a central switch for turning on biologically important cellular and viral genes, and demonstrate the complex pattern of viral gene expression in EBV-associated tumor cells. They do not provide, however, a definite answer to the question which role EBV might play in lymphomagenesis.

Viral Integration is a Feature Frequently Observed in EBV Positive Burkitt's Lymphoma Cells

In most Burkitt's lymphoma cell lines a third fragment of 177 b was protected, corresponding in size exactly to the part of the probe derived from exon 1. The RNA giving rise to the 177 b fragment should be alternatively spliced from the splice donor at the end of exon 1 to another exon than exon 2. This additional exon could be of either viral or cellular origin. A splice to cellular sequences is suggested by the fact that the 177 b fragment is also protected by RNA of Namalwa cells which are known to contain only two integrated but no episomal copies of the viral genome [5, 8]. Namalwa cells were reported not to harbor TP1 and TP2 mRNA [15] which is consistent with the absence of the 327 b and 150 b fragments in the S1 experiment with Namalwa RNA (fig. 2). The 177 b fragment was detected in all Burkitt's lymphoma lines expressing TP1 RNA. This suggests that integration of viral DNA into the host genome is a frequent, if not regular feature of Bur-

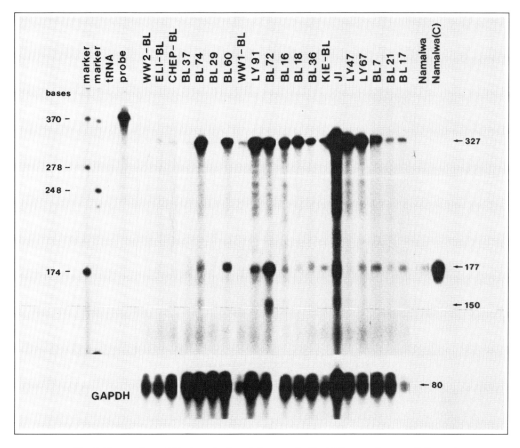

Fig. 2. Expression of the terminal protein gene in Burkitt's lymphoma cell lines. A M13 subclone of TP1 cDNA containing 177b of exon 1 and 150b of exon 2 was uniformly labelled and used for S1 analysis. Detection of glyceraldehyde-phosphate dehydrogenase (GAPDH) with a synthetic oligonucleotide served as internal standard.

kitt's lymphoma, and that both RNAs initiating at the same promoter are coordinately regulated.

The Role of EBV in Burkkitt's Lymphoma

With regard to the role of EBV in the development of Burkitt's lymphoma we are left with the following possibilities:

1. EBNA1 might be involved not only in episomal viral replication but also in providing a growth advantage to the tumor cell.

2. EBNA2 and other viral genes involved in the induction of lymphoproliferation play a role only in the initial stage of the development of the disease, but are not important for maintaining tumor cell growth. Alternatively, EBNA2 might be expressed and play a role at a very low level of expression.

3. Viral integration might lead to activation or inactivation of cellular genes involved in positive and negative regulation of cell growth, as suggested also for other human DNA viruses such as HBV and HPV.

4. Integration might render the TP gene independent of EBNA2 by inserting a cellular promoter in front of the coding part of TP2. It will be important to rule out the existence of such RNAs by more sensitive S1 analyses using poly A^+ RNA.

5. EBV might hide in Burkitt's lymphoma cells without providing a growth advantage to the tumor cell.

Conclusions

These studies have demonstrated the complexity of the pattern of EBV latent gene expression in neoplastic cells and stressed the importance of EBNA2 as an activator of viral and cellular genes. The analysis of TP expression has provided circumstancial evidence that integration of EBV DNA into the host genome is a common feature of Burkitt's lymphoma. Cloning of aberrant TP transcripts will allow to characterize the presumed viral-cellular fusion transcripts and will provide a tool to get access to the sites of integration within the host genome. Apparently, characterization of integration sites is the prerequisite to study whether cellular genes are affected by the integration and, if so, whether perturbation of such genes by viral integration contributes to the development of Burkitt's lymphoma.

References

1   Bornkamm GW, Hudewentz J, Freese UK, Zimber U: Deletion of the nontransforming Epstein-Barr virus strain P3HR-1 causes fusion of the large internal repeat to the DSL-Region. J Viol 1982;43:952–968.
2   Bornkamm GW, Polack A, Eick D: C-myc deregulation by chromosomal translocation in Burkitt's lymphoma, in Klein G (ed): Cellular oncogene activation. New York, Marcel Dekker, 1988, pp 233–273.

3 Calender A, Billaud M, Aubry JP, Banchereau J, Vuillaume M, Lenoir GM: Epstein-Barr virus (EBV) can turn on B-cell activation markers upon in-vitro infection of EBV-genome-negative B-lymphoma cells. Proc Natl Acad Sci USA 1987;84:8060–8064.

4 Cordier M, Calender A, Zimber U, Rousselet G, Pavlish O, Blanchereau J, Tursz T, Bornkamm GW, Lenoir GM: Stable transfection of Epstein-Barr virus (EBV) nuclear antigen 2 in lymphoma cells containing the EBV/P3HR-1 genome induces expression of B-cell activation molecules CR2 and CD23. J Virol (1990) in press.

5 Henderson A, Ripley S, Heller M, Kieff E: Chromosome site for Epstein-Barr virus DNA in a Burkitt tumor cell line and in lymphocytes growth-transformed in vitro. Proc Natl Acad Sci USA 1983;80:1987-1991.

6 Laux G, Perricaudet M, Farrell PJ: A spliced Epstein-Barr virus gene expressed in immortalized lymphocytes is created by circularization of the linear viral genome. EMBO J 1988;7:769–774.

7 Lenoir GM, Bornkamm GW: Burkitt's lymphoma, a human cancer model for the study of the multistep development of cancer: proposal for a new scenario. Adv Viral Oncol 1987;7:173–205.

8 Matsuo T, Heller M, Petti LO, Shiro E, Kieff E: Persistence of the entire Epstein-Barr virus genome integrated into human lymphocyte DNA. Science 1984;226:1322–1325.

9 Moss DJ, Misko IS, Burrows SR, Burman K, McCarthy R, Sculley TB: Cytotoxic T-cell clones discriminate between A- and B-type Epstein-Barr virus transformants. Nature 1988;331:719–721.

10 Mueller Lantzsch N, Lenoir GM, Sauter M, Takaki K, Bechet JM, Kuklik-Roos C, Bornkamm GW: Identification of the coding region for a second Epstein-Barr virus nuclear antigen (EBNA2) by transfection of cloned DNA fragments. EMBO J 1985; 4:1805–1811.

11 Murray RJ, Young LS, Calender A, Gregory CD, Rowe M, Lenoir GM, Rickinson AB: Different patterns of Epstein-Barr virus gene expression and of cytotoxic T-cell recognition in B-cell lines infected with transforming (B95-8) or nontransforming (P3HR-1) virus strains. J Virol 1988;62:894–901.

12 Rooney CM, Gregory CD, Rowe M, Finerty S, Edwards C, Rupani H, Rickinson AB: Endemic Burkitt lymphoma: Phenotypic analysis of tumor biopys cells and of derived tumor cell lines. J Natl Cancer Inst 1986;77:681–687.

13 Rowe DT, Rowe M, Evan GI, Wallace LE, Farrell PJ, Rickinson AB: Restricted expression of EBV latent genes and T-lymphocyte-detected membrane antigen in Burkitt's lymphoma cells. EMBO J 1986;5:2599–2607.

14 Rowe M, Rowe DT, Gregory CD, Young LS, Farrell PJ, Rupani H, Rickinson AB: Differences in B cell growth phenotype reflect novel patterns of Epstein-Barr virus latent gene expression in Burkitt's lymphoma cells. EMBO J 1987;6:2743–2751.

15 Sample J, Liebowitz D, Kieff E: Two related Epstein-Barr virus membrane proteins are encoded by separate genes. J Virol 1989;63:933–937.

U. Zimber-Strobl, Gesellschaft für Strahlen- und Umweltforschung mbH München, Institut für klinische Molekularbiologie und Tumorgenetik, Hämatologikum, Marchioninistraße 25, D-8000 München 70 (FRG)

Contrib Oncol, vol 39, pp 60–71 (Karger, Basel, 1990)

Molecular Characterization of the Chromosome 9q34 Breakpoint in Patients with t(6;9) Acute Non-Lymphocytic Leukemia (ANLL)

M. von Lindern[a], *S. van Baal*[a], *A. Poustka*[b] *and G. Grosveld*[a]

[a] Dept. of Cell Biology and Genetics, Erasmus University,
 Rotterdam, The Netherlands
[b] ZMBH, University of Heidelberg, FRG

A large number of lymphoid and myeloid leukemias are specified by defined chromosomal aberrations [1]. It has been put foreward that chromosome aberrations play an active role in the generation of leukemias [2–5]. However, only during the last decade tools became available to analyze and molecularly define these events. Our interest is focussed on the role of chromosome translocations in myeloid leukemias. During the last seven years, it was shown that protooncogenes located at or near chromosomal breakpoints of translocations are altered by this event. For the few cases analyzed to date, the translocation leads to expression of altered gene products and/or aberrant expression of normal gene products, that are directly involved in transformation of the relevant hematopoietic target cells (reviewed in [6]). Examples of such genes were found in B- and T-cell lymphomas, where proto-onocgenes were found to be translocated to immunoglobulin (IG-gene) and T-cell receptor (TCR) gene segments e. g.: Bcl-1, Bcl-2; Lyl-1; c-myc [7, 8]. Isolation of chromosomal breakpoints of B- and T-cell lymphomas has been relatively successful, since they could be detected and cloned with IG or TCR gene segment probes. This approach, however, was not applicable for the identification of chromosome translocations in myeloid leukemias, explaining why to date only one single myeloid chromosome translocation has been analyzed at the molecular level; the Philadelphia translocation in chronic myeloid leukemia (reviewed in [9]). To extend the knowledge on genes involved in myeloid leukemogenesis, we started a programm to molecularly characterize the (6;9) translocation in acute non-lymphocytic leukemia.

A relative rare subtype of ANLL (0.5 %) is characterized by the t(6;9) (p23;q34) and was first described by Rowley and Potter [10]. Patients with t(6;9) ANLL are relatively young, they present with ANLL of FAB-M2 (60 %), M4 (30 %) or even M1 and all respond poorly to therapy [11]. The specific occurrence of the t(6;9) suggests that the disruption or activation of one or more genes, located near the breakpoints on chromosome 6 or 9 is involved in the generation of this type of leukemia. Proto-oncogenes mapping in the vicinity of the chromosomal breakpoints on 6p23 and 9q34 are human pim-1 and c-ABL, respectively [12, 13]. Analysis of the pim-1 gene in t(6;9) ANLL showed that the gene is expressed at an elevated level in these patients, but the breakpoint is more than 165 kb away from the pim-1 gene [14]. This observation makes it unlikely that the pim-1 gene is transcriptionally activated by the translocation. Westbrook et al. [15] showed by *in situ* hybridization, that the c-ABL gene remains on chromosome 9 in two patients with t(6;9) ANLL. This observation was confirmed for a third case by von Lindern et al. [14], who analyzed the position of c-ABL in human/ hamster somatic cell hybrids, containing the segregated translocation chromosomes of a t(6;9) ANLL patient. From these studies it became clear that the 9q34 breakpoint in t(6;9) ANLL occurs telomeric from c-ABL. Moreover, long range mapping experiments showed that the breakpoint is more than 300 kb downstream of c-ABL [14].

Materials and Methods

Patients

Bone marrow of t(6;9) ANLL patients was obtained from several hospitals in Europe. DK, JK and SE were obtained from Amsterdam and Rotterdam, The Netherlands, PL from Leuven, Belgium and PM from Stockholm, Sweden. Cytogenetic analysis showed the presence of t(6;9) in all patients except for SE.

Libraries

The NotI jumping library was described by Poustka et al. [16]. The human chromosomal EMBL-3 and cosmid libraries were described by de Klein et al. [18] and Hermans et al. [19]. The K562 cDNA library was described by Domen et al. [20]. The human testis cDNA library was obtained from Clonetech, California, USA.

Field Inversion Gelelectrophoresis (FIGE)

FIGE was performed according to von Lindern et al. [14].

Results

Localization of the t(6;9) ANLL Breakpoint on Chromosome 9q34

In order to generate a probe far downstream (telomeric) from c-ABL (towards the (6;9) breakpoint) a NotI chromosome jumping library was screened [16] with a probe containing the c-ABL exon 1A sequences. As shown in figure 1, c-ABL is situated at the centromeric end of a 300 kb NotI fragment. Six independent phage clones were recovered and analyzed. All six clones contained the 0.5 kb NotI-BamHI c-Abl 1A exon fragment, the sup F tag plasmid and a new 1.6 kb BamHI-NotI fragment (fig. 1). Since the latter fragment was present in all clones, it most likely represented the telomeric end of the 300 kb NotI fragment. To verify this, probes from both ends of the jumping clone, 1A-NB and AJ1-R3 (fig. 1) were hybridized to a Southern blot, containing NotI digested DNA of Hela cells, separated by field inversion gelelectrophoresis (FIGE, 17). Both probes detected the same 300 kb Not fragment (fig. 1), indicating that the jumping clones indeed contained the telomeric end of the 300 kb NotI c-ABL fragment. Screening of a normal human genomic λ-library with probe AJ1-R3 (fig. 1) produced a λ-linking clone, from which probe AL1-BB, could be isolated (fig. 1). This probe hybridizes to the adjacent telomeric Not1 fragment. As shown in figure 1, the Not1 fragment measures 200 kb and is detected in DNA from a human/hamster hybrid cell line, containing the normal chromosome 9 from a t(6;9) ANLL patient (patient DK [14]). However, in the somatic cell hybrid containing the 9q+ derivitative of this patient, a 350 kb NotI fragment is detected by probe AL1-BB. This experiment indicated that the 200 kb NotI fragment could contain the chromosomal breakpoint of t(6;9) ANLL patient DK. To prove this point, standard chromosome walking experiments were started, to molecularly clone the 200 kb NotI fragment. For the walking experiments, human cosmid and λ-EMBL-3 libraries were used. At present 150 kb of the 200 kb NotI fragment has been obtained in overlapping clones. The EcoRI restriction map of this area is shown in figure 2. To verify, whether the 200 kb NotI fragment contains the t(6;9) ANLL breakpoints, DNA isolated from bone marrow of patients was ana-

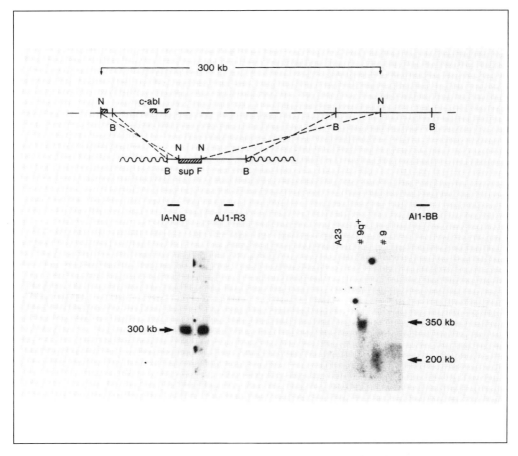

Fig. 1. Isolation of a NotI c-ABL jumping clone. The top part of the figure represents the 300 kb NotI fragment containing the human c-ABL gene at the left end (centromeric). The NotI site in the c-ABL 1A exon is indicated. The line beneath the map represents one of 6 λ jumping clones isolated from a NotI-BamHI jumping library. Besides the 0.5 kb NotI-BamHI c-ABL fragment and the sup F tag plasmid, these clones contained a 1.6 kb BamHI-NotI fragment representing the telomeric end of the 300 kb NotI fragment. Probes 1A-NB and AJ1-R3, indicated by the black horizontal bars beneath the jumping clone, detect a 300 kb fragment a FIGE-blot containing NotI digested HeLa cell DNA (bottom left part). Using probe AJ1-R3 a λ-linking clone was isolated (not shown) from which probe AL1-BB could be isolated (indicated at the top right part of the figure). As shown on the bottom right part of the figure, this probe detects a 200 kb NotI fragment on a FIGE blot containing DNA from a somatic cell hybrid containing normal human chromosome 9 († 9). A fragment of 350 kb is detected in NotI digested DNA of a hybrid cell line, containing chromosome 9q+ from a t(6;9) ANLL patient († 9q+). In hamster DNA (A23), no hybridizing fragments are detected. N = NotI, B= BamHI.

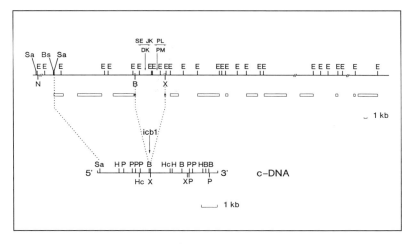

Fig. 2. Genomic and cDNA maps of the CAN-gene on chromosome 9q34. The top line represent the EcoRI restriction map of the CAN gene. At the left, the NotI site is indicated to which the NotI jump was made. The map between this NotI site and the BsshII site has been deleted (-//-). The distance between these two sites measures 30 kb. The SacII site coincides with the 5′-end of the CAN gene. The area bordered by the BamHI and XbaI sites represents the intron containing t(6;9) breakpoints; icb-1. Positions of the breakpoints of 5 t(6;9) ANLL patients (SE, DK, JK, PL, PM) in icb-1 are indicated above the map. Two regions of unknown size (-//-) at the 3′ side (telomeric) of the gene have not been isolated. The minimal size of the CAN gen is 120 kb. Open boxes beneath the map indicate genomic restriction fragments containing exon sequences. The bottom line represents the restriction map of the CAN cDNA. The transcriptional direction is indicated. Corresponding 'reference' sites; Sa, B, x, in the cDNA and the genomic DNA are indicated by dotted lines. B = BamHI, Bs = BsshII, E = EcoRI, H = HindIII, Hc = HincII, P = PstI, Sa = SacII, X = XbaI.

lyzed with several rare cutting restriction enzymes. A probe 30 kb downstream of the NotI site (to which the jump was made), recognizes a 180 kb BsshII fragment in control DNA (fig. 3, lanes 1 and 2). This fragment is comprised in the 200 kb NotI fragment and is also detected in the hybrid cell line containing human chromosome 9 (fig. 3, lane 6). Aberrant fragments of 150 kb are detected in DNA from bone marrow of two t(6;9) ANLL patients (lane 3, patient JK; lane 4, patient PL) and in DNA of a hybrid cell line containing the 9q+ chromosome of patient DK (lane 5). The 150 kb fragment in the sample of patient PL hybridizes weakly, because the bone marrow of this patient contains only 30 % blast cells [14]. It is noteworthy that the probe used in this experiment, cross-hybridizes to hamster DNA and detects a 150 kb hamster fragment in cell line A3 (fig. 3, lanes 6 and 7). The

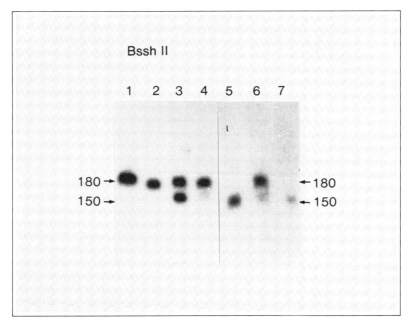

Fig. 3. Detection of 9q34 breakpoints in t(6;9) ANLL patients. DNA digested with BsshII was separated on a FIGE gel, blotted to nylon membrane and hybridized to a probe that maps 30 kb downstream from the NotI site isolated by chromosome jumping (fig. 1). Lane 1 and 2 contain normal human DNA; lane 3 and 4 DNA from bone marrow of 2 t(6;9) ANLL patients; lane 5 DNA from a hamster/human somatic cell hybrid containing a t(6;9) 9q+ chromosome; lane 6 DNA from a hybrid containing chromosome 9; lane 7 DNA of hamster cell line a23. The probe cross-hybridizes to a hamster NotI fragment of 150 kb. Numbers at the sides of the figure indicate the size of fragments in kb.

experiment shows, that the t(6;9) breakpoint on chromosome 9q34 of three patients is present in the 180 kb BsshII fragment.

Isolation of DNA Encompassing the 9q34 Breakpoint of t(6;9) ANLL

During the chromosome walking experiments, probes derived from newly generated clones were hybridizes to the panel of hamster hybrid cell lines, containing the segregated human t(6;9) chromosomes [14]. This procedure was used to test whether probes mapped on chromosome 9, or were translocated to the 6p- chromosome (not shown). Probes mapping 60 kb downstream from the NotI-site fulfilled this criterion. A physical map of this region is shown in figure 4, in which 2 probes F4EP and F6E3 are indicated. The two probes were hybridized to Southern blots, containing BamHI and BglII digests of DNA from the hybrid panel of patient DK and DNA from bone marrow of t(6;9) ANLL patients DK, JK, PL, PM and SE. In all 5 patients, aberrant restriction fragments show up by the combination

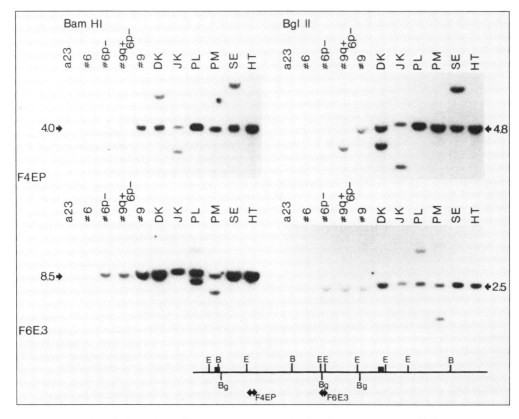

Fig. 4. Detection of chromosome 9 breakpoints in patients with t(6;9) ANLL. Southern blots of BamHI and BglII digested DNAs from a human/hamster hybrid panel containing human chromosome 6, 6p-, 9q+/6p- and 9 of t(6;9) ANLL patient DK and bone marrow DNA of patients DK, JK, PL, PM, SE, hybridized with probes F4EP and F6E3. These probes map 30 kb downstream form the BsshII site indicated in figure 4. Controls are hamster DNA, cell line a23 and normal human thymus DNA (HT). The map at the bottom of the figure shows the position of probes F4E (5′) and F6E3 (3′) (black arrows) in the icb-1 of t(6;9) ANLL patients. Small black boxes on this map indicate restriction fragments that cross-hybridize to cDNA probes. Numbers at the sides of the figure indicate the size of restriction enzyme fragments in kb.

of the two probes: F4EP detects aberrant BamHI and BglII fragments in patients DK, JK and SE, while F6E3 detects such fragments in patients PL and PM (fig. 4). Mapping of the breakpoint area shows that they occur in an stretch of 9 kb of DNA (fig. 2).

The Breakpoint Region of Chromosome 9q34 is Part of a Gene

The probe, cross-hybridizing to hamster DNA, was used to screen two λ-gt10 cDNA libraries, derived from the CML cell line K562 and adult human testis, respectively. The K562-library produced a 2 kb cDNA clone (not shown), that was used as a starting point for cDNA walking experiments. Repeated screening of the libraries yielded 5 overlapping cDNA clones, containing 7.5 kb cDNA sequences (not shown). The restriction map of the cDNA is shown in Figure 2. The transcriptional direction of the gene (fig. 2) was determined by the use of strand specific cDNA probes (not shown).

Hybridization of the 7.5 kb cDNA sequences to cloned genomic DNA identified 14 genomic fragments containing exon sequences, as indicated by open boxes in figure 2. The position of the BamHI and XbaI sites in the centre of the cDNA are also indicated in the genomic DNA (fig. 2). It is clear that the position of the 9q34 breakpoint of the 5 t(6;9) ANLL patients maps between the BamHI and XbaI sites on the genomic DNA. Since the distance between these two sites in the cDNA is 50 basepairs and in the genomic DNA 9 kb, the breakpoints map within an intron of 9 kb (fig. 2). Thus the (6;9) breakpoints map within an intron of a gene, situated telomeric from c-ABL on chromosome 9q34. We propose to call this gene CAIN (abbreviated CAN) and the *i*ntron *c*ontaing the *b*reakpoints, icb-1.

CAN Transcription in t(6;9) ANLL Patients

In order to study the influence of the 9q34 breakpoint on the transcription of the CAN-gene, cDNA probes mapping 5′ and 3′ of the 1cb-1 were used to hybridize to Northern blots, containing RNA from several human cell lines (Hela, Daudi, HSB, KG1, ML1, HL60 and K562) and bone marrow RNA from two t(6;9) ANLL patients (DK, SE). The 5′ as well as the 3′ probe detect a major 7.5 kb mRNA species in most cell lines and several minor larger mRNAs of unknown origin. However, in the patient samples, no mRNA is detected by the 5' cDNA probe (not shown) while the 3' probe detects a new 5.5 kb mRNA (fig. 5). The 3' part of the CAN-gene, that is translocated to the 6p- chromosome, encodes 4.2 kb of CAN mRNA (fig. 2). Therefore it is conceivable, that the 3' part (4.2 kb) of the new 5.5 kb mRNA molecule in these two t(6;9) ANLL patients consists of CAN-sequences while the 5' side of the mRNA (1.3 kb) is derived from sequences not present in the normal 7.5 kb CAN mRNA.

Discussion and Conclusions

Through the combination of longe range mapping, chromosome jumping and chromosome walking techniques, it appeared to be possible to clone the 9q34 breakpoint area (icb-1) of the specific t(6;9) chromosome translocation in ANLL. The tactics used to isolate the icb-1 on 9q34 can be used to isolate and identify any other chromosome translocation in human

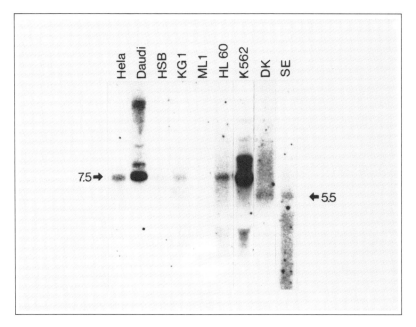

Fig. 5. CAN-mRNAs in cell lines and t(6;9) ANLL patients. A Northern blot containing RNA from human cell lines (Hela, Daudi, HSB, KG1, ML1, HL60 and K562) and two t(6;9) ANLL patients (DK, SE) was hybridized to cDNA sequences located 3' of the icb-1 (see fig. 4). The numbers at the sides of the figure indicate sizes of mRNAs in kb.

cancer. It is obvious however, that in the case described in this report, the conditions for successful isolation of the t(6;9) 9q34 breakpoints were favourable:

1. The starting probe (c-ABL exon 1A) was situated at the 5' end of a 300 kb NotI fragment and could immediately be used to screen the NotI chromosome jumping library.

2. Both the orientation of c-ABL gene on chromosome 9 was known as well as the relative position of the t(6;9) 9q34 breakpoints with respect to c-ABL.

The most striking feature of the breakpoint analysis in t(6;9) ANLL patients on 9q34 is, that in all 5 cases analyzed, the breakpoints map in a limited region of 9 kb, icb-1. Through cloning of the cDNA, it became clear that the icb-1 is part of a large gene that measures at minimum 120 kb. This gene, CAN is transcribed in telomeric direction (5' centromeric, 3' telomeric) on chromosome 9, identical to c-ABL. The icb-1 most likely represents an intron in the CAN-gene. Sequence analysis of the icb-1 region in the cDNA (fig. 2) and the corresponding exons in the genomic DNA will provide evidence whether the icb-1 indeed represents one entire intron. Experiments to investigate this question are now in progress.

The second interesting observation is provided by the Northern blot analysis of t(6;9) ANLL bone marrow RNA. Only CAN probes mapping at the 3' side of the icb-1 detect a new CAN-mRNA of 5.5 kb in patients, while in myeloid and lymphoid cell lines a major species of 7.5 kb is detected. Provided that the cloned cDNA sequences represent a full length copy of the 7.5 kb CAN mRNA, then the 3' part of the mRNA that is translocated to the 6p- chromosome measures 4.2 kb. However, the new CAN-mRNA measures 5.5 kb, indicating that 1.3 kb of this mRNA is encoded for by sequences not present in the normal CAN-mRNA. Several models could explain this observation of which two are mentioned:

1. Through the translocation event a cryptic promoter could be activated in the icb-1. The promoter would add 1.3 kb of 5' intronic sequences to the rest of the 4.2 kb CAN-mRNA, resulting in a new 5.5 kb CAN-mRNA.

2. Alternatively, the translocation may fuse the 3' part of the CAN-gene to the 5' part of a gene on chromosome 6. The chimeric gene would then be transcribed from a real or a cryptic promoter on chromosome 6. This configuration would result in a fusion mRNA that consists at its 5' side of 1.3 kb of chromosome 6 sequences spliced to 4.2 kb of CAN sequences.

Cloning of the cDNA of the 5.5 kb CAN mRNA present in these patients will define its exact nature and will distinguish between the two possibilities. The creation of a chimeric gene on the 6p- chromosome would resemble the fusion of the BCR and ABL gene on the Philadelphia chromosome in CML. As to the biological function of the CAN-gene within the cell, nothing is known at present.

The Northern blotting data show that expression of CAN is not restricted to myeloid cells (K562, ML1, HL60, KG1), but also occurs in cells of lymphoid an epithelial origin (Daudi, HSB, HeLa). Sequence analysis of the cDNA may reveal homologies to known nucleic acid or protein sequences, which may give insight in its possible function in the cell. It is unclear whether the translocation of the 3' part of the CAN gene to chromosome 6p- creates a truncated or fusion gene with oncogenic potential. Expression of cDNAs representing the 5.5 kb new CAN mRNA in suitable cell lines and/or transgenic mice will show whether this gene has transforming potential. The specificity of the translocation breakpoints within the CAN-gene and the formation of a new CAN mRNA in t(6;9) ANLL patients strongly argues for an active role of this translocation in the genesis of this subtype of ANLL.

Acknowledgements

We thank Dr. D. Bootsma for continuous support and discussion; Drs. F. Mitelman, A. Hagemeijer, H. Adriaansen, C. Mecucci, H. van den Berghe, D. Veerman for patient material; R. Boucke and M. Kuit for preparation of the manuscript and photographic work. This work is supported by the Dutch Cancer Foundation (Koningin Wilhelmina Fonds).

References

1   Yunis JJ, Soreng AL, Bowe AE: Fragile sites are targets of diverse mutagens and carcinogens. Oncogene 1987;1:59–70.
2   Nowel PC, Hungerford DA: A minute chromosome in human chronic granulocytic leukemia. Science 1960;132:1497.
3   Sandberg A, Kohno SI, Wake N, Minowada J: Chromosomes and causation of human cancer and leukemia XLII. Cancer Genet Cytogenet 1980;2:145–174.
4   Rowley JD: Identification of the constant chromosome regions involved in human hematologic malignant disease. Science 1982;216:749–751.
5   Mitelman F: Restricted number of chromosomal regions implicated in aetiology of human cancer and leukemia. Nature 1984;310:325–327.
6   Cory S: Activation of cellular oncogenes in hematopoietic cells by chromosome translocation. Adv Cancer Res 1986;47:189–234.

7   Croce CM: Role of chromosome translocations in human neoplasia. Cell 1987;
     49:155–156.
8   Mellentin JD, Smith SD, Cleary ML: Lyl-1, a novel gene altered by chromosomal
     translocation in T-cell leukemia, codes for a protein with a helix-loop-helix DNA
     binding motif. Cell 1989;58:77–83.
9   Kurzrock R, Gutterman JK, Talpaz M: The moleclular genetics of Philadelphia chro-
     mosome-positive leukemias. New Engl J Med 1988;13:990–998.
10   Rowley JD, Potter D: Chromosomal banding patterns in acute non-lymphocytic leu-
     kemia. Blood 1976;47:705–721.
11   Heim S, Kristofferson U, Mandahl N, Mitelman F, Benhassy AN, Genwicz S, Wiebe
     T: High resolution banding analysis of the reciprocal translocation t(6;9) in acute
     non-lymphocytic leukemia. Cancer Genet Cytogenet 1986;22:195–201.
12   Ngarajan L, Louie E, Tsujimoto Y, Ar-Rushdi A, Huebren K, Croce CM: Localiza-
     tion of the pim oncogene (Pim) to a region of chromosome 6 involved in transloca-
     tions in acute leukemias. Proc Natl Acad Sci USA 1986;83:2556–2560.
13   De Klein A, Geurts van Kessel A, Grosveld G, Bartram CR, Hagemeijer A, Bootsma
     D, Spurr NK, Heisterkamp N, Groffen J, Stephenson JR: A cellular oncogene is trans-
     located to the Philadelphia chromosome in chronic myelocytic leukemia. Nature
     1982;300:765–767.
14   Von Lindern M, van Agthoven T, Hagemeijer A, Adriaansen H, Grosveld G: The
     human pim-1 gene is not directly activated by the translocation (6;9) in acute non-
     lymphocytic leukemia. Oncogene 1989;4:75–79.
15   Westbrock CA, Le Beau MM, Diaz MO, Groffen J, Rowley JB: Chromosomal locali-
     zation and characterization of c-abl in the t(6;9) of acute nonlymphocytic leukemia.
     Proc Natl Acad Sci USA 1985;82:8742–8746.
16   Poustka A, Pohl TM, Barlow DP, Frischauf AM, Lehrach H: Construction and use of
     human chromosome jumping libraries from NotI digested DNA. Nature 1987;
     325:353–355.
17   Carle CF, Fank M, Olsen MV: Electrophoretic separations of large DNA molecules
     by periodic inversion of the electric field. Science 1986;232:65–68.
18   De Klein A, van Agthoven T, Groffen J, Heisterkamp N, Groffen J, Grosveld G:
     Molecular analysis of both translocation products of a Philadelphia-positive CML
     patient. Nucl Acid Res 1986;14:7071–7081.
19   Hermans A, Selleri L, Gow J, Wiedemann L, Grosveld G: Molecular analysis of
     the Philadelphia translocation in chronic myelogenous and acute lymphoblastic leu-
     kemia in Cancer cells, molecular diagnostics of human cancer. Cold Spring Harbor
     Laboratory Press 1989, vol 7, pp 21–26.
20   Domen J, von Lindern M, Hermans A, Breuer M, Grosveld G, Berns A: Comparison
     of the human and mouse Pim-1 cDNAs; nucleotide sequence and immunological
     identification of the *in vitro* synthesized Pim-1 protein. Oncogene Res 1987;1:103–
     112.

G. Grosveld, Dept. of Cell Biology & Genetics, Erasmus University,
P.O. Box 1738, 3000 DR Rotterdam (The Netherlands)

Contrib Oncol, vol 39, pp 72–85 (Karger, Basel, 1990)

Transgenic Window on Haematopoietic Neoplasia

J. M. Adams, A. W. Harris, D. L. Vaux, W. S. Alexander, H. Rosenbaum, S. P. Klinken, A. Strasser, M. L. Bath, S. Cory

The Walter and Eliza Hall Institute of Medical Research, Royal Melbourne Hospital, Victoria, Australia

Transgenic mice bearing oncogenes provide a valuable new tool for dissecting the multi-step process of neoplastic transformation [1]. To obtain insights into the genetic basis of haemopoietic neoplasia, we have constructed a series of transgenic lines harbouring different oncogenes suspected to play a role in the aetiology of lymphomas or leukaemias. In order to target expression to the haemopoietic cells, the genes were linked to the immunoglobulin heavy chain enhancer, which can function not only in B cells also in T cells and certain myeloid cells [2, 3]. The oncogenes studied represent different classes. Two encode the nuclear oncoproteins *myc* and N-*myc*, while two others encode related cytoplasmic tyrosine kinases: v-*abl* and a gene, *bcr*-v-*abl*, that mimics the hybrid gene formed in chronic myeloid leukaemia. Another, a mutant N-ras gene, encodes a cytoplasmic GTPase thought to transduce a growth factor signal, while the *bcl*-2 gene specifies a cytoplasmic protein of unknown function.

Mice bearing these genes exhibit a strong, heritable predisposition to specific types of tumours (table 1), but the sporadic fashion in which the malignant clones appear suggests that other events, presumably genetic, contribute to tumour development. We will first describe our findings with each of the transgenic strains, and then outline observations on how certain of the genes may interact and an approach for identifying novel cooperating oncogenes.

Table 1. Transgenic strains predisposed to haemopoieic neoplasia

Strain	Vector	Preneoplastic effects	Tumour types	References
Eμ-*myc*	[natural]*	pre-B cell overproduction	Pre-B, B	[4–6]
Eμ-N-*myc*	EμSV	pre-B cell overproduction	Pre-B	[7]
Eμ-v-*abl*	EμSV	none yet observed	plasmacytomas** lymphomas**	[34]
Eμ-*bcr*-v-*abl*	EμV$_H$	none yet observed[+]	pre-B, T	[8]
LTR-*bcr*-v-*abl*	LTR	none yet observed[+]	T	[8]
Eμ-N-*ras*	EμSV	none yet observed[++]	T, macrophage[++]	
Eμ-*bcl*-2	EμSV	B cell overproduction		[35]

* Complete *myc* gene and its promoters, essentially as found in one plasmacytoma [4].
** Three strains develop plasmacytomas and the other develops lymphomas.
[+] Lines examined showed no preneoplastic expression of the gene [8].
[++] Harris et al., in preparation.

Models for Specific Haematological Neoplasms

B-Lymphomagenesis Provoked by *myc* and N-*myc*

Young healthy Eμ-*myc* mice contain no transplantable malignant cells, but their pre-B and B cells are uniformly large and most [perhaps all] are in cycle [6]. Thus, constitutive c-*myc* expression may prevent B lymphoid cells from entering the G$_0$ state. The process of B lymphoid differentiation in the mice is clearly abnormal, because pre-B cells are elevated 4- to 5-fold and Ig-bearing cells slightly depressed (fig. 1). Moreover, although the mice are immunocompetent, fewer Ig-bearing cells respond immunologically, perhaps because the cells are not fully mature [9]. We therefore proposed that c-*myc* expression regulates the balance between self-renewal and differentiation, constitutive expression promoting self-renewal at the expense of maturation but not imposing a complete block on differentiation [6].

Since *myc* is considered a nuclear transducer of signals from growth factor receptors, it is somewhat surprising that the growth properties of preneoplastic Eμ-*myc* pre-B cells are very similar to those of normal pre-B cells. In liquid culture, they die rapidly unless provided with a stromal feeder layer [10], and they fail to grow as colonies in agar [11, 12]. Thus the cells appear to retain their absolute dependence on growth factors and do not appear to be immortal, despite the commonly held notion that *myc* is an

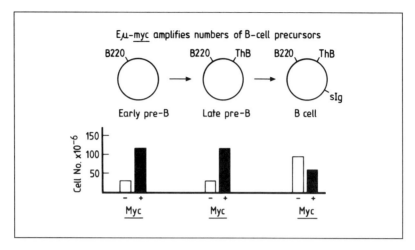

Fig. 1. Constitutive *myc* expression perturbs B cell development. The numbers of cells at three stage of B lineage development were evaluated by flow cytometry using the indicated cell surface markers [6]. Results for Eμ-*myc* mice (solid bars) are compared with those from nontransgenic littermates (unfilled bars).

immortalising gene. Nevertheless, as in the transgenic mice, the Eμ-*myc* lymphocytes growing on feeder layers are large and at least 2.5 times as many as normal are in cycle. Thus the *myc*-driven cells appear either to remain in cycle or to die [10].

After about six weeks of age, clonal pre-B or B lymphomas begin to develop among the Eμ-*myc* mice [4, 5]. The kinetics of tumour onset suggests that the rate at which the cycling, benign pre-B cells spontaneously convert to malignancy is about 10^{-10} per cell division [5]. It is thus possible that the tumorigenic process requires more than one somatic mutation. Indeed, in vitro, at least two stages were apparent. After prolonged culture on stromal cells (14–20 weeks), Eμ-*myc* pre-B cells started to grow to 10-fold higher densities but were not tumorigenic; eventually, a tumorigenic clone emerged [10].

Somatic alteration of the *myc* transgene could be invoked as a step contributing to tumorigenesis. In human Burkitt lymphomas, *myc* exon 1 mutations have been implicated in tumorigenesis, since the *myc* gene has not only been translocated to an immunoglobulin locus but usually also mutated near the 3′ border of exon 1 [13], a region were *myc* transcription is attenuated [14] and translation of a larger *myc* polypeptide initiates [15]. To determine whether exon 1 mutations are necessary, we utilised the polymerase chain reaction to analyse *myc* mRNA sequences from the exon 1 region in five E*μ-myc* B lymphoid tumours [16]. None were found; hence exon 1 alteration is not necessary to render *myc* tumorigenic. Moreover, no structural rearrangement of the E*μ-myc* gene could be detected in any of 20 tumours and in only two cases was there any amplification. We conclude [16] that somatic mutation of the E*μ-myc* transgene is unlikely to account for the onset of tumours in E*μ-myc* mice.

On the hypothesis that tumour onset requires activation of an independent oncogene, we screened 14 E*μ-myc* lymphoma DNAs for genes capable of transforming NIH-3T3 fibroblasts to grow as fibrosarcomas in nude mice. Fibrosarcomas with a particularly rapid onset were provoked by DNA from two lymphomas. These lymphomas were found to carry a mutated N-*ras* or K-*ras* gene [17], the mutation in each case involving amino acid 61, one of the three residues most frequently implicated in *ras* activation [18]. The mutated N-*ras* gene was cloned into a retroviral vector and shown to transform pre-B cells from E*μ-myc* mouse bone marrow [17]. Thus a spontaneous *ras* mutation contributed to the development of two of the E*μ-myc* tumours, but the collaborating genes responsible for the majority of the tumours do not register in the fibroblast assay and remain to be identified. The relevant genes might prove to include anti-oncogenes as well as oncogenes.

N-*myc* has been associated primarily with neuroblastoma and small cell lung carcinoma, and its expression within the B lineage is normally confined to the earliest maturation stages [19], unlike *myc*, which is expressed in almost all dividing cells. Nevertheless, we found that its enforced expression throughout the B lymphocyte compartment gave effects very similar to *myc* [7]. The E*μ*-N-*myc* mice succumbed to clonal pre-B or B cell lymphomas at rates comparable to those of E*μ-myc* mice, and the bone marrow of the pre-lymphomatous mice contained an elevated level of cycling pre-B cells. Other recent evidence suggests that N-*myc* may also be lymphomagenic for T cells (eg. 20). It is noteworthy, however, that the N-*myc* transgene is expressed at a level much higher than normal for the endogenous N-*myc* gene [7], whereas E*μ-myc* espression is comparable to that in normal proliferating B cells [21]. Thus, N-*myc* may be oncogenic only when grossly overexpressed, whereas even modest overexpression of *myc* may suffice.

As shown previously for the c-*myc* gene [4, 21], N-*myc* appears to be subject to negative feedback regulation. The endogenous N-*myc* and c-*myc* alleles are silent in the E*μ*-N-*myc* pre-B lymphomas [7]. Moreover, the silence of the c-*myc* gene in these tumours argues that N-*myc* can completely supplant *myc* function in cell proliferation and that N-*myc* can regulate c-*myc* expression. Since the endogenous N-*myc* as well as c-*myc* alleles are silent in Eμ-*myc* pre-B lymphomas [7], N-*myc* and c-*myc* appear to be subject to cross-regulation as well as autoregulation. Alt and his colleagues have reached similar conclusions from independently developed Eμ-N-*myc* mice [22].

V-*abl* Provokes Plasmacytomas Harbouring *myc* Rearrangements

Abelson murine leukaemia virus, which bears the v-*abl* oncogene, can generate pre-B and T lymphomas and accelerate development of plasmacytomas in BALB/c mice also treated with the mineral oil pristane, but its effects are strongly influenced by the route of virus administration and the helper virus used [23]. To study the impact of v-*abl* on lymphoid cells in the absence of such complicating variables, we developed several strains of mice carrying the *gag-abl* gene from Abelson virus linked to the SV40 promoter and IgH enhancer (Eμ-v-*abl* strains). Although their lympho-haemopoietic development was apparently normal, three strains proved to have a remarkable predisposition to develop plasmacytomas (Rosenbaum et al. [34]). Strikingly, at least 80 % of the plasmacytomas contained a rearranged c-*myc* gene and half of these seemed to result from linkage of *myc* to the immunoglobulin Cα gene. These data strongly suggest that v-*abl* and *myc* co-operate in the transformation of plasma cells. Indeed, the rate-limiting step for the onset of Eμ-v-*abl* plasmacytomas may well be the chance of a *myc* translocation occurring in a single member of the susceptible population. Our data complement earlier observations [24] that the plasmacytomas induced by Abelson virus in pristane-treated BALB/c mice carry *myc* translocations.

In view of the predilection of Abelson virus for pre-B lymphomagenesis why have no lymphomas appeared in three independent Eμ-v-*abl* lines? The transgene is clearly capable of generating such tumours, because they do arise in a fourth Eμ-v-*abl* line under study. As illustrated in Fig. 2, the hypothesis we favour to reconcile this paradox is that v-*abl* induction of pre-B lymphomas requires its activity within a very early cell type, one that is infectable by Abelson virus but in which the IgH enhancer, and hence an Eμ-transgene, is usually inactive (Presumably the transgene in the lymphoma-prone Eμ-v-*abl* line is activated abnormally early by some influence of the flanking DNA). The model posits that the typical Abelson virus pre-B lymphoma results from continued differentiation of the transformed cell,

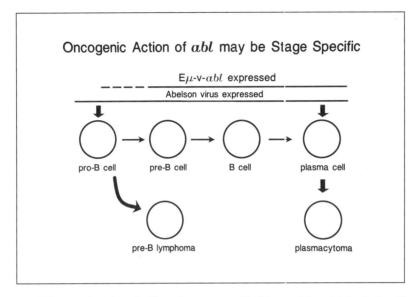

Fig. 2. Oncogenic action of *abl* may be stage specific. The model postulates that v-*abl* oncogenesis is confined to the plasma cell and a primitive lymphoid progenitor. The Abelson virus can infect all stages, but the Eμ-driven transgene will usually be silent at the earlier stage.

at least with respect to IgH rearrangement (see below). Recent data generated with sorted cell populations also suggest that the major Abelson target is more primitive than the pre-B cell [25].

Lymphomas Elicited by *bcr*-v-*abl*

A *bcr-abl* fusion gene is associated with both chronic myeloid leukaemia (CML) and some cases of acute lymphoblastic leukaemia (ALL). To test the effects of *bcr-abl* on haemopoetic cells, we constructed a *bcr*-v-*abl* gene that mimics the CML translocation product [26]. When delivered by a retrovirus to a factor-dependent myeloid cell line, the synthetic gene, like *bcr*-c-*abl*, could render the cells autonomous [26]. To study effects in vivo, we made transgenic mice having *bcr*-v-*abl* coupled to the immunoglobulin enhancer or, in an attempt to promote myeloid expression, to the enhancer and promoter from the long terminal repeat of myeloproliferative sarcoma virus (table 1).

Unexpectedly, both transgenes elicited only lymphoid tumours [8]. T lymphomas predominated, but the Eμ-*bcr*-v-*abl* mice also developed some pre-B lymphomas. Curiously, only a minority of the mice initially studied developed tumours, and the transgenes did not appear to be expressed in the non-tumourous animals [8]. Subsequent breeding of one Eμ-*bcr*-v-*abl* line, however, has yielded a line in which lymphomas consistently arise at a very young age. Thus an expressed *bcr*-v-*abl* gene may be remarkably potent in vivo, at least within the lymphoid lineage. Developing a transgenic animal model for CML may be difficult, however, because that may require targetting expression to the haemopoietic stem cell without inducing embryonic lethality.

N-*ras* Provokes T Lymphomas and Macrophage Tumours, But No B Lymphomas

Although a mutated *ras* gene, most frequently N-*ras*, is common in certain forms of leukaemia, its aetiological role remains problematic, because the mutation is often not present in all the leukaemic cells [18]. To establish that a mutant *ras* gene could initiate haemopoietic tumours, we developed two strains of mice bearing an Eμ-N-*ras* gene with an aspartate at codon 12. To our surprise, no mice from either line have developed any B lymphoid tumours, despite evidence of transgene expression in B lymphoid cells (see below). They become ill instead with thymic T lymphomas and/or histocytic sarcomas, which reside predominantly in the spleen and liver and appear to be of macrophage origin [Harris et al, in preparation]. These unexpected observations suggest that a mutant N-*ras* gene can initiate tumour development much more effectively in T lymphoid cells or macrophages than in B lymphoid cells. Curiously, N-*ras* expression has not promoted any obvious alteration in lympho-hematopoietic development.

Bcl-2 Provokes an Excess B Cell Syndrome

The *bcl*-2 gene was discovered by virtue of its fusion to the IgH locus in human follicular cell lymphomas carrying the 14;18 chromosome translocation [27]. While clearly a candidate oncogene, the biological activity of *bcl*-2 was unknown. The first clue to its function was our observation [28] that immortal but factor-dependent cell lines infected with a *bcl*-2-bearing retrovirus remained viable after removal of growth factor, although they did not proliferate. This finding suggested that *bcl*-2 represents a novel type of oncogene that confers a survival advantage rather than a proliferative function.

To explore the oncogenic potential of *bcl*-2 and characterise its activity in vivo, we developed strains of mice expressing *bcl*-2 under the control of the IgH enhancer and either an SV40 or V_H promoter [35]. Intriguingly, spleen cells from such mice also exhibit the ability to survive exposure to adverse growth conditions: when plated in vitro in medium containing serum but no lymphokines, the transgenic cells survived far longer than cells from normal littermates. Korsmeyer and his colleagues also observed this phenomenon in their strains of *bcl*-2 transgenic mice [29]. Our *bcl*-2 mice exhibit limited splenomegaly, increased numbers of lymphocytes in the peripheral blood and an increased frequency of sIg^+B lymphoid cells in haemopoietic tissues, particularly the bone marrow. The small size of these cells suggests that they are not actively proliferating. The data from *bcl*-2 mice are consistent with the hypothesis that constitutive *bcl*-2 expression confers on the typical G_0 lymphocyte a greatly increased lifespan in vivo, presumably because the cell is now resistant to conditions (such as a dearth of factors) that normally promote its demise. Thus one role of *bcl*-2 in oncogenesis may simply be to promote the longevity of the B lymphocyte clone bearing the 14;18 translocation and hence increase its chance of acquiring another activated oncogene [28], or of forfeiting an anti-oncogene. Significantly, sporadic haemopoietic tumours are beginning to occur in the Eμ-*bcl*-2 colony.

Myc Synergy with Known Oncogenes

Although the need for more than one genetic event to render a normal cell tumorigenic is now widely accepted, most of the evidence derives from in vitro studies with a few fibroblastic cell types, and much less has been established for very different cell types, such as haemopoietic cells. Our studies illustrate how several types of genes work together with the *myc* gene to promote haemopoietic neoplasia. For example, lymphoma development was greatly accelerated when newborn Eμ-*myc* mice were infected with a helper-free retrovirus bearing the v-H-*ras* or the v-*raf* oncogene [30]. Moreover, infection of bone marrow cells in vitro with either virus allowed many transgenic cells to grow autonomously, to clone in agar and to generate tumours in nude mice [11, 12]. Hence an activated *ras* or *raf* gene can collude with *myc* in B lymphoid transformation. Further striking evidence of ras/*myc* cooperativity was provided when the Eμ-*myc* and Eμ-N-ras mice were bred. The 'doubly transgenic' progeny developed tumours within the first few weeks of life and, remarkably, all were derived from early B lineage tumours [Harris et al, in preparation]. Despite this clear evidence of *myc*/*ras* synergy, it remains an open question whether *myc* plus *ras* is sufficient to transform a lymphocyte immediately or whether another genetic alteration ensues.

Notable albeit less dramatic synergy was observed in vitro between *bcl*-2 and *myc*. Infection of Eμ-*myc* bone marrow cells with a *bcl*-2 virus allowed very slow outgrowth of cell lines, several of which eventually became tumorigenic [28]. Thus the *bcl*-2/*myc* combination seems to promote immortalization but does not itself produce an autonomous clone. That is not surprising, since neither gene alone nor the combination appears to replace the proliferative stimulus provided by the cognate growth factor [28].

Oncogenic cooperation between v-*abl* and *myc* may be confined to certain maturation stage. Despite the elevated level of pre-B cells in Eμ-*myc* mice, infection of the newborn animals with helper-free Abelson virus did not accelerate the formation of pre-B lymphomas, although one plasmacytoma developed [30]. Similarly, no synergy could be discerned in transformation of Eμ-*myc* bone marrow cells in vitro [11, 12]. At the plasma cell stage, on the other hand, the evidence that most plasmacytomas of Eμ-v-*abl* mice bear *myc* translocations (see above) strongly suggests that the two genes act in concert, as was verified when mice bearing both transgenes developed very rapid, oligoclonal plasmacytomas (Rosenbaum et al. [34]). The issue of whether *myc* plus v-*abl* can transform every plasma cell remains unresolved, but an attractive possibility is that proliferation of particular clones of cells expressing the two genes is favoured by antigenic stimulation.

Detection of Cooperating Oncogenes by Insertional Mutagenesis

Since retroviruses that lack an oncogene can contribute to tumourigenesis by chance insertion near critical cellular genes, we are exploiting Moloney leukaemia virus to identify genes able to collaborate with deregulated *myc* expression. This approach has been used by Berns and his colleagues [20] to identify genes which accelerate T lymphoma onset in transgenic mice harbouring *pim*-1, a gene frequently implicated in the development of T lymphomas. Strikingly, Eμ-*myc* mice infected as newborns with Moloney virus were moribund before uninfected transgenic littermates became ill (fig. 3). As the tumours were B lymphoid, whereas this virus produces only T cell tumours in conventional mice, they must have arisen by synergy between Eμ-*myc* expression and Moloney virus insertion.

To screen the virus-induced Eμ-*myc* tumours for proviral insertion near a collaborating oncogene, tumour DNAs were first analysed for rearrangement of oncogenes known to contribute to lymphoid tumourigenesis, e.g. *cbl, bcl*-2, *pim*-1, *raf* and *abl*. Somewhat surprisingly, a substantial proportion (19 %) of the B lymphomas bear proviruses near *pim*-1. Thus, *pim*-1 can contribute to B as well as T cell neoplasia. A second approach has been to determine whether any proviral insertion sites are common to several tumours. Already one such site has been identified (our unpublished results). The DNA flanking a provirus cloned from one tumour proved to be rearranged in at least 27 % of the other tumours. This locus, which we have provisionally designated *bmi*-1 [*B* lymphoma *M*oloney virus *i*nsertion region-1], is transcribed at higher levels in the tumours harbouring a rearrangement than in those that lack one. The *bmi*-1 gene, which has also been detected by A. Berns and Colleagues, is being characterised by cloning and sequencing *bmi*-1 cDNA. This analysis will clarify its relationship to c-*bic* [31], a proviral insertion region recently implicated as collaborators with *myc* in avian B lymphoid tumours.

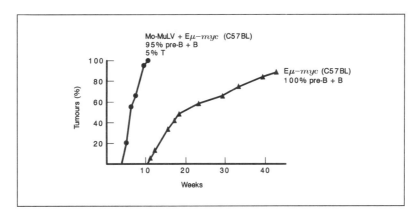

Fig. 3. Acceleration of lymphomagenesis in Eμ-*myc* mice by infection with Moloney leukaemia virus.

Puzzles and Prospects

As well as confirming in a prospective fashion the oncogenic character of genes previously implicated in haemopoietic neoplasia, the novel tumour-prone strains (table 1) are helping to clarify the pathways to malignancy. Already it is evident that the transgenes affect lymphocyte development in very different ways. Constitutive *myc* or N-*myc* expression elicits an expanded pool of cycling pre-B cells, whereas *bcl*-2 produces an elevated level of resting B cells. These results are consonant with the notion that the products of *myc* genes discourage the cell from entering G_0 [6, 7], whereas *bcl*-2 promotes cellular longevity [28]. Curiously, despite the high predisposition of the other transgenic strains to develop tumours, no alteration in lymphocyte development has yet been observed. Hence tumour predisposition need not involve a hyperplastic state.

Some puzzles are also raised by the predisposition to particular tumour types (table 1). Since *myc* has long been implicated in T lymphoma development [32], their absence in *myc* and N-*myc* lines may merely reflect low T cell expression for those lines [7, 21], or it may be related to genetic background, since an Eμ-*myc* transgene has given T lymphomas in C3H mice [33]. For v-*abl*, we have suggested above that oncogenic activity is confined to two stages of B lymphoid development (fig. 2). For *bcr*-v-*abl*, we suspect that the absence of myeloid effects is due to lack of expression in the most relevant target: the haemopoietic stem cell. For the N-*ras* oncogene, we cannot as yet offer a satisfactory explanation for the absence of B lineage tumours, since *myc* activation obviously can overcome this deficiency, but the results seem to hint that the order of acquisition of two oncogenes can affect the outcome.

To date our attempts to identify the event(s) responsible for emergence of the tumorigenic clone have met with greatest success for the v-*abl* plasmacytomas, where *myc* translocations are the culpable agents, while *ras* mutation plays a minor role in the Eμ-*myc* lymphomas. The dramatic evidence of *myc/ras* synergy in lymphoma onset suggests that much may be learned from crosses of some of the other transgenic strains. Moreover, the insertional mutagenesis approach has already revealed that not only a known locus (*pim*-1) but also an apparently novel one (*bmi*) can collaborate with *myc* in B lymphoma development. This general approach should be applicable to any of the other strains. It may well provide access to previously unknown genes that contribute to tumour development.

Acknowledgments

Our research is supported by The National Health and Medical Research Council (Canberra) and the U.S. National Cancer Insitute (CA43540 and CA12421). We thank Wally Langdon, Iswar Hariharan, Elizabeth Webb and Judy McNeall for their participation in several of the studies cited here.

References

1   Cory S, Adams JM: Transgenic mice and oncogenesis. Ann Rev Immunol 1988; 6:25–48.
2   Kemp DJ, Harris AW, Cory S, Adams JM: Expression of the immunoglobulin $C\mu$ gene in mouse T and B lymphoid and myeloid cell lines. Proc Natl Acad Sci USA 1980;77:2876–2880.
3   Grosschedl R, Weaver D, Baltimore D, Constantini F: Introduction of a μ immunoglobulin gene into the mouse germ line: specific expression in lymphoid cells and synthesis of functional antibody. Cell 1984;38:647–658.
4   Adams JM, Harris AW, Pinkert CA, Corcoran LM, Alexander WS, Cory S, Palmiter RD, Brinster RL: The c-*myc* oncogene driven by immunoglobulin enhancers induces lymphoid malignancy in transgenic mice. Nature 1985;318:533–538.
5   Harris AW, Pinkert CA, Crawford M, Langdon WY, Brinster RL, Adams JM: The $E\mu$-*myc* transgenic mouse: a model for high-incidence spontaneous lymphoma and leukemia of early B cells. J Exp Med 1988;137:353–371.
6   Langdon WY, Harris AW, Cory S, Adams JM: The c-*myc* oncogene perturbs B lymphocyte development in $E\mu$-*myc* transgenic mice. Cell 1986;47:11–18.
7   Rosenbaum H, Webb E, Adams JM, Cory S, Harris AW: N-*myc* transgene promotes B lymphoid proliferation, elicits lymphomas and reveals cross-regulation with c-*myc*. EMBO J 1989;8:749–755.
8   Hariharan IK, Harris AW, Crawford M, Abud H, Webb E, Cory S, Adams JM: *Bcr-v-abl* oncogene induces lymphomas in transgenic mice. Mol Cell Biol 1989;9:2798–2805.
9   Vaux DL, Adams JM, Alexander WS, Pike B: Immunologic competence of B cells subjected to constitutive c-*myc* expression in immunoglobulin heavy chain enhancer *myc* transgenic mice. J Immunol 1989;179:3854–3860.
10 Langdon WY, Harris AW, Cory S: Growth of $E\mu$-*myc* transgenic B-lymphoid cells in vitro and their evolution towards autonomy. Oncogene Res 1988;3:271–279.
11 Dyall-Smith D, Cory S: Transformation of bone marrow cells from $E\mu$-*myc* transgenic mice by Abelson murine leukemia virus and Harvey murine sarcoma virus. Oncogene Res 1988;2:403–409.
12 Alexander WS, Adams JM, Cory S: Oncogene co-operation in lymphocyte transformation: malignant conversion of $E\mu$-*myc* transgenic pre-B cells in vitro by v-H-*ras* or v-*raf* but not v-*abl*. Mol Cell Biol 1989;9:67–73.
13 Pelicci P-G, Knowles DM, Magrath I, Dalla-Favera R: Chromosomal breakpoints and structural alterations of the c-*myc* locus differ in endemic and sporadic forms of Burkitt lymphoma. Proc Natl Acad Sci USA 1986;83:2984–2988.

14 Bentley DL, Groudine M: Sequence requirements for premature termination of transcription in the human c-*myc* gene. Cell 1988; 53:245–256.

15 Hann SR, King MW, Bentley DL, Anderson CW, Eisenman RN: A non-AUG translational initiation codon in c-*myc* exon 1 generates an N-terminally distinct protein whose synthesis is disrupted in Burkitt's lymphomas. Cell 1988;52:185–195.

16 Webb E, Barri G, Cory S, Adams JM: Lymphomagenesis in Eµ-*myc* transgenic mice does not require transgene rearrangement or mutation of *myc* exon 1. Mol Biol Med 1989;6:475–480.

17 Alexander WS, Bernard O, Cory S, Adams JM: Lymphomagenesis in Eµ-*myc* transgenic mice can involve *ras* mutations. Oncogene 1989; 4:575–581.

18 Bos JL: Ras oncogenes in human cancer: a review. Cancer Res 1989;49:4682–4689.

19 Zimmerman KA, Yancopoulos GD, Collum RG, Smith RK, Kohl NE, Dennis KA, Nau MM, Witte ON, Toran-Allerand D, Gee CE, Minna JD, Alt FW: Differential expression of *myc* family genes during murine development. Nature 1986;319:780–783.

20 Van Lohuizen M, Verbeek S, Krimpenfort P, Domen J, Saris C, Radaszkiewicz T, Berns A: Predisposition to lymphomagenesis in *pim*-1 transgenic mice: cooperation with c-*myc* and N-*myc* in murine leukemia virus-induced tumours. Cell 1989;56:673–682.

21 Alexander WS, Schrader JW, Adams JM: Expression of the c-*myc* oncogene under control of an immunoglobulin enhancer in Eµ-*myc* transgenic mice. Mol Cell Biol 1987;7:1436–1444.

22 Dildrop R, Ma A, Zimmerman K, Hsu E, Tesfaye A, DePinho R, Alt FW: IgH enhancer mediated deregulation of N-*myc* gene expression in transgenic mice: generation of lymphoid neoplasias that lack c-*myc* expression. EMBO J 1989;8:1121–1128.

23 Whitlock CA, Witte ON: The complexity of virus-cell interactions in Abelson virus infection of lymphoid and other hematopoietic cells. Adv Immunol 1985;37:73–98.

24 Ohno S, Migita S, Wiener F, Babonits M, Klein G, Mushinski JF, Potter M: Chromosomal translocations activating *myc* sequences and transduction of v-*abl* are crucial events in the rapid induction of plasmacytomas by pristane and Abelson virus. J Exp Med 1984;159:1762–1777.

25 Tidmarsh GF, Heimfeld S, Whitlock CA, Weissman IL, Muller-Sieburg: Identification of a novel bone marrow-derived B-cell progenitor population that coexpresses B220 and Thy-1 and is highly enriched for Abelson leukemia virus targets. Mol Cell Biol 1989;9:2665–2671.

26 Hariharan IK, Adams JM, Cory S: *bcr*-v-*abl* oncogene renders myeloid line factor independent: potential autocrine mechanism in chronic myeloid leukemia. Oncogene Res 1988;3:387–399.

27 Tsujimoto Y, Finger LR, Yunis J, Nowell PC, Croce, CM: Cloning of the chromosome breakpoint of neoplastic B cells with the t[14;18] chromosome translocation. Science 1987;226:1097–1099.

28 Vaux DL, Cory S, Adams JM: *Bcl*-2 gene promotes haemopoietic cell survival and cooperates with c-*myc* to immortalize pre-B cells. Nature 1988;335:440–442.

29 McDonnell TJ, Deane N, Platt FM, Nunez G, Jaeger U, McKearn JP, Korsmeyer SJ: *bcl*-2-immunoglobulin transgenic mice demonstrate extended B cell survival and follicular lymphoproliferation. Cell 1989;57:79–88.

30 Langdon WY, Harris AW, Cory S: Acceleration of B lymphoid tumourigenesis in Eμ-*myc* transgenic mice by v-H-*ras* and v-*raf* but not v-*abl*. Oncogene Res 1989; 4:253–258.

31 Clurman BE, Hayward WS: Multiple proto-oncogene activation in avian leukosis virus-induced lymphomas: evidence for stage-specific events. Mol Cell Biol 1989; 9:2657–2664.

32 Corcoran LM, Adams JM, Dunn AR, Cory S: Murine T lymphomas in which the cellular *myc* oncogene has been activated by retroviral insertion. Cell 1984;37:113–122.

33 Yukawa K, Kikutani H, Inomot T, Uehira M, Bin SH, Akagi K, Yamamura K-I and Kishimoto T: Strain dependency of B and T lymphoma development in immunoglobulin heavy chain enhancer (Eμ)-*myc* transgenic mice. J Exp Med 1989;170:711–726.

34 Rosenbaum H, Harris AW, Bath ML, McNeall J, Webb E, Adams JM, Cory S: An Eμ-v-*abl* transgene elicits plasmacytomas in concert with an activated *myc* gene. EMBO J 1990;9:897–905.

35 Strasser A, Harris AW, Vaux DL, Webb E, Bath ML, Adams JM, Cory S: Abnormalities of the Immune System Induced by Dysregulated *bcl*-2 Expression in Transgenic Mice. Curr Topics Microbiol Immunol [in press].

J.M. Adams, The Walter and Eliza Hall Institute of Medical Research, Post Office Royal Melbourne Hospital, Victoria, 3050 (Australia)

Contrib Oncol, vol 39, pp 86–93 (Karger, Basel, 1990)

Molecular Events During Tumor Progression in Neuroblastoma

R. Bernards[a], *M. Lenardo*[b]

[a] Department of Molecular Genetics, The Cancer Center of the Massachusetts
  General Hospital and Harvard Medical School, Charlestown, MA
[b] Laboratory of Immunology, National Institute for
  Arthritis and Infectious Disease, National Institues of Health, Bethesda,
  MD, USA

The N-myc oncogene was fist identified as an amplified DNA element with homology to c-*myc* in human neuroblastoma [1, 2]. Since this initial observation, amplification of N-*myc* has also been observed in other types of human cancer, predominantly in retinoblastoma and small cell lung cancer [3, 4]. The apparent role of the N-*myc* oncogene in neuroblastoma oncogenesis is unusual in that amplification of N-*myc* is hardy ever observed in primary non-metastatic neuoblastoma. Rather, amplification of N-*myc* has been found predominantly in advanced, widely metastatic neuroblastoma [5, 6]. This close association between N-*myc* amplification and metastatic ability suggests that a relationship exists between these two phenomena, namely that N-*myc* over-expression is responsible for the increased metastatic ability of the N-*myc*-amplified tumor cells. The role of N-*myc* in neuroblastoma thus appears to be quite different from its role in other types of tumors, in which N-*myc* expression is thought to be an early event in the process of cell transformation. For instance, N-*myc* has been found to be frequently activated by proviral insertion in murine T-cell lymphomas [7], suggesting that transcriptional deregulation of N-*myc* is an early event in the genesis of T-cell lymphomas. Consistent with this latter notion, in vitro experiments have indicated thath the N-*myc* gene can immortalize primary rat embryo fibroblasts in tissue culture. Taken together, these data suggest that N-*myc* plays a role early in the process of oncogenic transformation, causing the transformation of a cell with limited in vitro lifespan into one that is immortal [8].

Our research has focused on understanding the mechanism by which the N-*myc* gene contributes to the increased metastatic ability of N-*myc*-amplified neuroblastomas, the results of which are discussed below.

N-myc as a Regulator of Cellular Gene Expression

The N-*myc* oncogene has been shown to encode a nuclear phosphoprotein that has the ability to bind to DNA [9]. These properties of the N-*myc* protein suggest that it might exert its oncogenic effect by deregulating the expression of certain key cellular genes, the altered expression of which is responsible for the N-*myc*-induced changes in cellular behavior. Thus, N-*myc* over-expression in neuroblastoma may cause an alteration in the expression of cellular genes which leads to increased metastatic ability. We have attempted to identify cellular genes whose expression is affected by N-*myc* in neuroblastoma in an attempt to find an explanation at the molecular level for the increased metastatic ability of N-*myc*-amplified neuroblastoma tumor cells.

To identify genes whose expression is altered in neuroblastoma by N-*myc* we followed up on an observation made earlier regarding the mechanism of adenovirus-mediated transformation. In this system, we found that the E1A oncogene of the highly oncogenic adenovirus type 12 was able to suppress the expression of the major histocompatibility compley (MHC) class I antigens in transformed cells [10]. Since MHC class I antigens are required for the recognition of foreign antigens by cytotoxic T-lymphocytes [11], their absence from the surface of adenovirus 12-transformed cells explained why these cells could induce tumors in immunocompetent hosts.

To investigate whether the N-*myc* oncogene shared the ability of the adenovirus E1A oncogene to suppress the expression of the MHC class I antigens, we screened a number of human neuroblastoma tumor cell lines for their expression of both MHC class I antigens and N-*myc*. We found that in all cell lines tested the expression of N-*myc* was inversely correlated with the expression of MHC class I antigens [121]. Although these experiments suggested that there might be a relationship between the expression of N-*myc* and MHC class I in neuroblastoma, these initial observations did not prove that a causal relationship existed between the expression patterns of these two genes.

To further study the possible relationship between the expression of N-*myc* and MHC class I, we used a rat neuroblastoma cell line named B104. These rat cells resembled human neuroblastoma which did not carry an amplified N-*myc* gene in that they grew slowly but progressively in immunocompetent rats without progressing to form metastases. By transfecting an N-*myc* expression vector into B104 cells, we obtained a series of N-*myc* expressing derivatives of this parental cell line. The N-*myc*-transfected derivatives were found to have undergone several major changes in phenotype. First, the N-*myc*-transfected derivatives of the B104 cell line were strikingly more malignant: following injection in immunocompetent syngeneic rats, N-*myc*-transfected B104 cells grew rapidly and formed widespread metastases. In this respect, the N-*myc*-transfected B104 cells seemed to resemble advanced childhood neuroblastoma in which over-expression of N-*myc* is also associated with increased metastatic ability [5, 6]. Significantly, N-*myc*-transfected B104 cells were also found to have a substantial decrease in the expression of MHC class I antigens, indicating that N-*myc* was indeed responsible for the low MHC class I phenotype of neuroblastomas [12].

Mechanism of Transcription Regulation by N-myc

The experiments described above supported the long-standing hypothesis that *myc* oncogenes could act to deregulate cellular gene expression. It therefore appeared of considerable interest to us to investigate in detail the mechanism by which the N-*myc* gene product could modulate the expression of MHC class I antigens.

To do this, we first investigated whether N-*myc* acted to suppress the transcription of MHC class I antigens in neuroblastoma cells. We found that the murine MHC class I H-2K^b promoter was approximatelly 10- to 15-fold less active in B104 N-*myc*-transfected cells as compared to the parental B104 cells, indicating that N-*myc* acted to suppress MHC class I at the level of transcription initiation [13]. By analyzing the activity of a series of deletion mutants from this murine H-2K^b promoter construct in both B104 and B104 N-*myc*-transfected cells, we found that one of the major sites on which N-*myc* acted to suppress MHC class I antigen expression was an enhancer element centered around nucleotide-166 of the murine H-2K^b promoter [13]. This enhancer had previously been shown to stimulate the activity of the MHC class I gene promoter [14].

Furthermore, it had been shown that this enhancer element stimulated transcription through the binding of a nuclear factor, named H2TF1 [14]. These results suggested the possibility that N-*myc* suppressed the activity of this enhancer element by interfering with the binding of this nuclear factor to the MHC class I gene enhancer.

To investigate this, we prepared nuclear extracts from B104 neuroblastoma cells and its N-*myc*-transfected derivatives and tested these in a gel electrophoresis DNA-binding assay with an oligonucleotide corresponding to the MHC class I gene enhancer as a probe. The results of this experiment, shown in figure 1a, indicate that B104 neuroblastoma cells contain a nuclear protein that binds to the wild-type MHC class I gene enhancer (lane B104-wt), but not to a mutant version of this element (lane B104-M). Significantly however, B104 N-*myc*-transfected cells were found to contain much lower levels of this nuclear factor. Reduced binding of nuclear factor to the MHC class I gene enhancer in the N-*myc*-transfected cells did not appear to be caused by proteolytic degradation of the nuclear extract, since the same extract contained high levels of nuclear factor binding to the immunoglobulin $\varkappa$E2 or μE3 binding sites (fig. 1b). Since this initial observation, we have also shown that N-*myc* markedly abrogates the binding of nuclear factors to the MHC class I gene enhancer in human neuroblastoma [13]. We conclude from these experiments that N-*myc* suppresses the expression of MHC class I genes by decreasing the binding of a nuclear factor to MHC class I gene enhancer, thereby functionally inactivating this element of the MHC class I gene promoter. The further study of the interaction between the N-*myc* oncoprotein and the H2TF1 transcription factor could yield important insights into the mechanism by which N-*myc* acts to deregulate cellular gene expression.

Neural Cell Adhesion Molecule Expression in Neuroblastoma Cells

The experiments described above established the N-*myc* gene product as a critical regulator of cellular gene expression. However, it appeared unlikely to us that in neuroblastoma N-*myc* would only affect the expression of MHC class I antigens. We therefore investigated the pattern of expression of several other genes, whose altered expression could potentially contribute to the increased metastatic ability of N-*myc* amplified neuroblastomas. One of the genes that we explored was the gene encoding neural cell adhesion molecule (NCAM), a family of related cell surface glycoproteins involved in cell-cell recognition and cell-cell adhesion.

Evidence that reduced NCAM expression could be relevant to the induction of metastatic ability comes from the study of NCAM expression

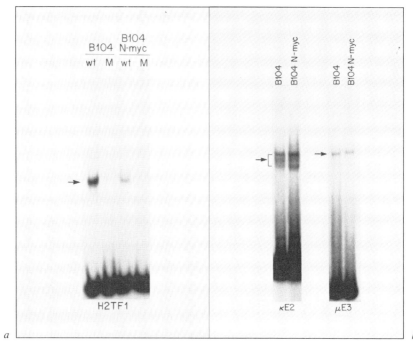

Fig. 1. Abundance of nuclear factors in neuroblastoma cells. Nuclear extracts were prepared from B104 neuroblastoma cells and N-*myc*-transfected B104 cells. Binding of nuclear factors was detected using a gel electrophoresis DNA-binding assay. *a.* 4000 cpm of ^{32}P-labeled oligonucleotide specifying either the consensus H2TF1-binding sequence (lanes indicated wt) or mutant H2TF1 sequence (lanes indicated M) was incubated with a nuclear cell extract from either B104 cells or B104 N-*myc*-transfected cells and separated on 4 % polyacrylamide gel. *b.* 4000 cpm of a DNA fragment specifying the binding site for either nuclear factor NF-*x*E2 or NF-*μ*E3 [18] was incubated with a nuclear extract as indicated and separated on a 4 % polyacrylamide gel.

during embryogenesis. Here it was found that premigratory neural crest cells, which are clustered adjacent to the dorsal neural tube, express readily detectable levels of NCAM polypeptides. However, as the cells leave this site to migrate towards the periphery as single cells, they do not express immunologically detectable NCAM. Upon arriving at their final anatomic location in the embryo they re-express NCAM [15]. Thus, migratory potential and NCAM expression are inversely related in neural crest cells. Since neural crest cells and neuroblastoma tumor cells are both derived from the neuro-ectodermal lineage, we felt it was possible that alterations in cell adhesion also contribute to the migratory potential of neuroblastoma tumor cells.

To investigate this, we measured NCAM levels in both B104 neuroblastoma cells and B104 N-*myc*-transfected cells. We found that several independently derived transfectants of the B104 neuroblastoma cell line that expressed N-*myc* at a high level had lost to a significant extent the expression of NCAM polypeptides and mRNA. A number of other neural components were not specifically suppressed by N-*myc*. Our data further indicate that revertants of the high N-*myc* phenotype that had lost most of their N-*myc* expression had regained significant levels of NCAM polypeptides, indicating that the continued expresion of N-*myc* was required to maintain the low levels of NCAM expression [16].

Conclusions

We have used a rat model system to study the effects of N-*myc* amplification on the malignancy of neuroblastoma tumor cells. Our data indicate that over-expression of N-*myc* in neuroblastoma tumor cells has at least three major effects. First, the rate at which N-*myc*-amplified tumor cells grow *in vivo* is greatly accelerated. In our rat B104 tumor system, we found that N-*myc* expressing neuroblastoma cells grew within 14 days to yield a tumor that was 300-fold larger in size than the tumor induced by the parental neuroblastoma cells. Second, we found that expression of N-*myc* leads to a dramatic reduction in the expression of MHC class I antigens, rendering the N-*myc*-amplified tumor cells resistant to T-cell-mediated immune destruction. Third, our data indicate that N-*myc* has the ability to suppress the expression of neural cell adhesion molecule. Since NCAM allows neuronal cells to adhere to each other, one would expect that neuroblastoma tumor cells that express reduced levels of these adhesion molecules have less of a tendency to adhere to the primary tumor mass than their non N-*myc*-amplified counterparts. N-*myc*-amplified neuroblastoma tumor cells may therefore break away from the primary site of tumor growth more readily than the non N-*myc*-amplified tumor cells, thus contributing to the increased metastatic ability of N-*myc*-amplified tumor cells. In support of this view is the recent finding that a highly metastatic subclone from a mouse melanoma cell line expressed much lower levels of NCAM than the parental low metastatic melanoma [17]. During their journey from the primary site of tumor growth to the secondary site, N-*myc*-amplified tumor cells should be protected from attack by cytotoxic T-lymphocytes due to the paucity of MHC class I antigens on these cells. Finally, the dramatically accelerated growth rate should help the N-*myc*-amplified tumor cells to proliferate at the secondary site to form a metastasis.

There is no doubt that the scenario described above represents an oversimplification of the events that take place during tumor cell metastasis. For instance, we have ignored the need for tumor cells to invade barriers such as the basement membrane and blood vessel walls. Nevertheless we feel that the observations made in the rat model system may very well begin to explain the differences in metastatic ability between non N-*myc*-amplified neuroblastomas and their N-*myc*-amplified counterparts. Molecular biology provides us with the tools to experimentally modulate the expression of MHC class I antigens and NCAM polypeptides in neuroblastoma cells. This should allow us to investigate the contribution of the altered expression of these cellular genes to the metastatic phenotype of neuroblastoma tumor cells in more detail.

Acknowledgments

The work described here was supported in part by grants from the Edward J. Mallinckrodt Foundation and the Searle Scholarship Foundation.

References

1   Schwab M, Altialo K, Klempnauer KH, Varmus HE, Bishop JM, Gilbert F, Brodeur G, Goldstein M, Trent J: Amplified DNA with limited homology to myc cellular oncogene is shared by human neuroblastoma cell lines and a neuroblastoma tumor. Nature 1983;305:245–248.
2   Kohl NE, Kanda N, Schreck RR, Bruns G, Latt SA, Gilbert F, Alt F: Transposition and amplification of oncogene related sequences in human neuroblastoma. Cell 1983;35:359–367.
3   Wong AJ, Ruppert JM, Eggleston J, Hamilton SR, Baylin SB, Vogelstein B: Gene amplification of c-myc and N-myc in small cell carcinoma of the lung. Science 1986; 233:461–464.
4   Lee WH, Murphee AL, Benedict WF: Expression and amplification of the N-myc gene in primary retinoblastoma. Nature 1984;309:458–460.
5   Brodeur GM, Seeger RC, Schwab M, Varmus HE, Bishop JM: Amplification of N-myc in untreated human neuroblastoma correlates with advanced stages of disease. Science 1984;224:1121–1124.

6   Seeger RC, Brodeur GM, Sather H, Dalton A, Siegel SE, wong KY, Hammond D:
     Associaton of multiple copies of the N-myc oncogene with rapid progression of neu-
     roblastoma. New Eng J Med 1985;313:1111–1116.
7   Van Lohuizen M, Breuer M, Berns A: N-myc is frequently activated by proviral inser-
     tion in MuLV-induced T cell lymphomas. EMBO J 1989;8:133–136.
8   Schwab M, Bishop JM: Sustained expression of the human oncogene MYCN rescues
     rat embryo cells from senescence. Proc Natl Acad Sci USA 1988;85:9585–9589.
9   Ramsay G, Stanton L, Schwab M, Bishop JM: Human proto-oncogene N-myc enco-
     des nuclear proteins that bind DNA. Mol Cell Biol 1986;6:4450–4457.
10   Schrier PI, Bernards R, Vaessen RTMJ, Houweling A, Van der Eb AJ: Expression of
     class I histocompatibility antigens switched off by highly oncogenic adenovirus 12 in
     transformed rat cells. Nature 1983;305:771–775.
11   Zinkernagel RM, Doherty PC: MHC-restricted cytotoxic T-cells: studies on the bio-
     logical role of polymorphic major transplantation antigens determining T-cell restric-
     tion-specificity, function, and responsiveness. Adv Immunol 1979;27:51–77.
12   Bernards R, Dessain SK, Weinberg RA: N-myc amplification causes down-modula-
     tion of MHC class I antigen expression in neuroblastoma. Cell 1986;47:667–674.
13   Lenaord M, Rustgi AK, Schievella AR, Bernards R: Suppression of MHC Class I
     gene expression by N-myc through enhancer inactivation. EMBO J 1989;8:3351–
     3355.
14   Baldwin ΛS, Sharp PA: Binding of a nuclear factor to a regulatory sequence in the
     promoter of the Mouse H-2K^b class I major histocompatibility gene. Mol Cell Biol
     1987;7:305–313.
15   Thierry JP, Duband JL, Rutishauser U, Edelman GM: Cell adhesion molecules in
     early chicken embryogenesis. Proc Natl Acad Sci USA 1982;79:6737–6741.
16   Akeson R, Bernards R: N-*myc* downregulates NCAM expression in rat neuroblas-
     toma Mol Cell Biol 1990;10:2012–2016.
17   Linneman D, Raz A, Bock E: Differential expression of cell adhesion molecules in
     variants of K1735 melanoma cells differing in metastatic capacity. Int J Cancer 1989;
     43:709–712.
18   Lenardo M, Pierce JW, Baltimore D: Protein-binding sites in Ig gene enhancers
     determine transcriptional activity and inducitbility. Science 1987;236:1573–1577.

R. Bernards, Ph. D., Department of Molecular Genetics,
The Cancer Center of the Massachusetts General Hospital
and Harvard Medical School,
143 13th Street, Charlestown, MA, 02129 (USA)

Contrib Oncol, vol 39, pp 94–114 (Karger, Basel, 1990)

The Transforming Growth Factor β Family of Growth Regulatory Peptides

R. W. Pelton, H. L. Moses

Department of Cell Biology, Vanderbilt University Medical School, Nashville, TN, USA

It has been widely postulated that processes such as cell proliferation, differentiation, morphogenesis and migration, which occur during normal embryonic development, as well as the factors which control these processes, may be reiterated, in an abberant fashion, during neoplasia. Indeed, tumor-derived cell lines are often used to study embryonic events and a large number of proto-oncogenes have now been found to be expressed during development [1] while their virally transformed counterparts are known to be active in carcinogenesis [2]. A large body of data now indicates that peptide growth factors are involved in both developmental as well as in neoplastic events. Perhaps no other growth factor can better serve to illustrate this observation than transforming growth factor β (TGFβ) and its family of related proteins. This family, which at present contains at least 14 members, has been shown to have a multitude of effects on cells of both embryonic and neoplastic origin. Based on sequence similarity, the family can be divided into a closely related group and a more distantly related group (see table 1). The purpose of this review is to give an overview of the TGFβ family and to briefly summarize the data suggesting a role(s) for the closely related members of the TGFβ family in embryogenesis with the obvious implication that many of these same processes may be involved in neoplasia. Until very recently, purified protein has been available only for TGFβ1 and TGFβ2, therefore studies done with these proteins will be emphasized. Where relevant, other members of the family will be discussed.

General Chemical Structure of the TGFβ Family

The term 'transforming growth factor' was derived from the ability of the first isolated family member, TGFβ1, to cause normal rodent fibro-

Table 1. The TGFβ family of genes

Gene	Class of origin	Biological activities of protein product
Closely-related-group		
TGFβ1	mammalian avian	inhibition of cell proliferation. Stimulation of connective and supporting tissue formation.
TGFβ2	mammalian	very similar to TGFβ1 with *in vitro* assays; more active in mesoderm induction in Xenopus.
TGFβ3	mammalian	similar to TGFβ1 and TGFβ2 in stimulating growth of fibroblasts and inhibiting growth of epithelial cells *in vitro*.
TGFβ4	avian	unknown.
Distantly-related-group		
MIS	mammalian	causes regression of Müllerian duct system in males.
Inhibin α Inhibin βA Inhibin βB	mammalian	the derived proteins, inhibins & activins, inhibit or stimulate FSH secretion by pituitary cells, respectively.
BMP-2a BMP-2b BMP-3	mammalian	induce ectopic cartilage formation *in vivo*
Vgr-1	mammalian	unknown.
Vg-1	amphibian	unknown. Thought to be involved in mesoderm induction.
XTC-MIF*	amphibian	mesoderm induction in Xenopus.
DPP	insectan	unknown. Null alleles give complete ventralization of embryo.

BMP, bone morphogenetic protein; DPP, Drosophila decapentaplegic; MIF, mesoderm in-ducing factor; MIS, Müllerian inhibiting substance; TGF, transforming growth factor.

*sequence data indicates that this is probably one of the inhibins.

blasts to take on a reversible transformed phenotype [3, 4]. Since TGFβ1 was the first member of the family to be isolated and characterized, it is considered the prototype molecule and hence the sequence similarity of subsequent family members has been reported relative to TGFβ1 (for a more complete review on the structure of the TGFβ family see [5] or [6]). Mature TGFβ1 is a 25 kD homodimeric protein composed of two 12.5 kD monomers linked by disulfide bonds. Sequence data has revealed that each monomer is synthesized as a 390 amino acid pre-pro-TGFβ1 (see fig. 1) and includes a 29 amino acid signal sequence which is cleaved to yield pro-TGFβ1 [7]. Pro-TGFβ1 consists of a 249 amino acid N-terminal glycopeptide (the precursor region) and a 112 amino acid C-terminal mature protein. The 112 amino acid mature region, comprising monomeric TGFβ1, is released from the precursor region at a dibasic cleavage site and dimerizes via cysteine-cysteine bonds to give mature TGFβ1. A general finding appears to be that secreted TGFβ1 is an inactive (latent) form. While it has long been known that extremes of pH can activate latent TGFβ1, recent evidence indicates that plasmin, a serine protease, may be a more physiological TGFβ1 activator [8, 9].

Within the TGFβ family, the region of highest sequence similarity is found in the carboxy-terminal portion of the molecule; this is the region in TGFβ1 which gives rise to the 112 amino acid mature protein. The closely-related members of the TGFβ family are TGFβ1 [10], TGFβ2 [11], TGFβ3 [6, 12], and TGFβ4 [13]. Sequence data indicates that the TGFβs 2–4 are all processed in a manner very similar to TGFβ1 (although TGFβ4 lacks a signal peptide) and release a mature monomer of 112–114 amino acids in length. While this mature carboxy-terminal region in the closely-related group shows amino acid sequence similarity on the order of 70–80 % (see table 2), with 9 of 9 cysteines invariably conserved, the N-terminal glycopeptide regions of these molecules are much less conserved. Comparison of amino acid sequence among various species has shown that within the 112 amino acid mature region of TGFβ1, human, bovine, and porcine TGFβ1 show 100 % sequence identity [14, 15]. The murine TGFβ1 differs by only 1 amino acid [16]. This amazing conservation of sequence identity

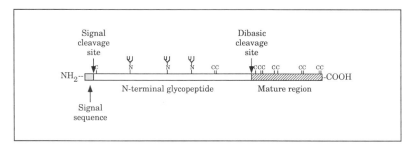

Fig. 1. A schematic representation of the pre-pro-TGFβ monomer. Shown are the signal sequence with its cleavage site, the N-terminal glycopeptide with its N-linked glycosylation sites and dibasic cleavage site, and the mature region of the molecule with its 9 cysteine residues.

across species boundaries suggests that the mature TGFβ1 molecule plays some critical role in the organism.

The distantly-related members of the TGFβ family include Müllerian inhibiting substance (MIS) [17], the inhibins α, βA, and βB [18], the bone morphogenetic proteins (BMPs) 2a, 2b and 3 [19], Vg-1 [20], Vgr-1 [21], and the decapentaplegic (DPP) gene product [22]. Sequence analysis of the members of the distantly-related group indicates that these molecules are more closely related to each other than to the TGFβs 1 – 4 (table 2). Indeed, sequence comparisons have shown that six members of the distantly-related group, the BMPs, Vg-1, Vgr-1, and DPP, comprise a distinct sub-group of which DPP is the prototype member [21]. By analogy to the closely-related group, the members of the distantly-related group show the highest sequence similarity in the C-terminal end of the molecule with 7 of the 9 cysteine residues invariably conserved. In addition, with the exception of MIS, all of the distantly-related members have basic residues preceding the highly conserved C-terminal region which could act as sites for proteolytic cleavage. However, at present, among the distantly-related group only the inhibins are known to be cleaved.

TGFβ Cell-Surface Receptors

Affinity cross-linking studies have demonstrated that TGFβ binds three structurally distinct cell surface receptors in a wide variety of normal and transformed cells of both epithelial as well as mesenchymal origin [23]. These receptors, which number from 2×10^3 to 4×10^4 per cell depending on the cell type, demonstrate dissociation constants on the order of 25 – 140 pM. All three receptors are glycosylated and they have been classified as type I (60 – 70 kD), type II (85 – 95 kD), and type III (280 – 330 kD) receptors [24 – 29]. The type III receptor, the predominant form found on most cells, appears to bind TGFβ1 and TGFβ2 with equal affinity, while the type I and type II receptors exhibit a tenfold higher affinity for TGFβ1 than for TGFβ2 [30]. Although it is at present unclear what roles each of these receptors play in the transduction of the TGFβ signal to the cell, studies of cells with mutant or absent type I receptors indicate that the type I receptor confers TGFβ sensitivity to the cell [23, 31]. It has been postulated that, by analogy to the IGF-I binding protein, perhaps the type II and type III receptors act as binding proteins which modulate the presentation of the ligand to the type I receptor.

Table 2. Polypeptide sequence identities (listed as percent) of the C-terminal (mature region) for 12 of the TGFβ family members after aligning for maximal homology. The origins are as follows: TGFβ1, TGFβ2, TGFβ3, MIS, Inhibin α, Inhibin βA, Inhibin βB, BMP-2a, BMP-2b are all from human; BMP-3 from bovine, Vg-1 from mouse, Vgr-1 from *Xenopus*, and DPP from *Drosophila*

	DPP	Vg-1	Vgr-1	BMP-3	BMP-2b	BMP-2a	Inhibin βB	Inhibin βA	Inhibin α	MIS	TGFβ3	TGFβ2
TGFβ1	35	31	34	32	38	37	33	42	27	31	77	72
TGFβ2	39	34	33	32	37	36	38	41	27	26	79	
TGFβ3	37	36	35	31	38	39	42	38	23	27		
MIS	30	34	24	31	33	30	26	27	25			
Inhibin α	22	23	21	34	23	24	25	26				
Inhibin βA	40	41	45	34	41	42	67					
Inhibin βB	40	40	38	38	42	42						
BMP-2a	71	62	61	48	87							
BMP-2b	73	60	59	48								
BMP-3	46	47	44									
Vgr-1	57	59										
Vg-1	50											

The post-receptor signaling mechanism employed by TGFβ receptors to give a biological response remains elusive. Studies indicate that the receptors possess no tyrosine kinase activity [32] or Na^+/H^+ antiport activity [33] nor have there been any reports of changes in the levels of inositol phosphate or intracellular Ca^{+2} following TGFβ binding. However, recent studies have shown that following TGFβ1 treatment of mouse fibroblasts, these cells demonstrate an increase in GTPase activity as well as an increase in GTPτS binding [34, 35]. In addition, Howe et al. [35] have shown that mink lung cells made insensitive to TGFβ1 following mutagenesis exhibit neither an increase in GTPase activity nor an increase in GTPτS binding. Hence, the data implicate G proteins in the transduction of the TGFβ signal through its receptors. In support of this, studies in which an activated H-*ras*, a G protein-related molecule, was transfected into cells indicate that these *ras*-transformed cells behave as though they are under continuous TGFβ treatment even though they do not produce increased levels of TGFβ [36].

Finally, it should be noted that of the members of the TGFβ family for which purified proteins have been obtained, only TGFβ1, TGFβ2 and TGFβ3 have been shown to bind to the type I, II, and III receptors. Interestingly TGFβ receptors have been found to be expressed by differentiated murine embryonal carcinoma cells [37]. Characterization of the receptors for MIS and the inhibins has not been reported.

TGFβ Effects on Cell Proliferation

The differences in effects of TGFβ1 and TGFβ2 on cell proliferation appear to be only quantitative and not qualitative. These effects are remarkably diverse and complex and are dependent not only on the cell type and culture conditions but on the general growth factor milieu as well [38]. Nonetheless, as a general rule it appears that TGFβ1 and TGFβ2 are mitogenic only for fibroblasts [39] and osteoblasts [40, 41], both cells of mesenchymal origin. Recently, TGFβ3 was also shown to be stimulatory to mouse fibroblasts [42].

The monolayer mitogenic effects of TGFβ1 differ from those seen to result from stimulation by other growth factors. This difference is both quantitative and qualitative inasmuch as both the degree and kinetics of the effects are different. Studies by Leof et al. [43] suggest that the stimulatory effects of TGFβ1 on mouse embryo fibroblasts are indirect and are due to

TGFβ1 induced PDGF synthesis. TGFβ1 treated fibroblasts showed an early induction mRNA for the proto-oncogene c-*sis* followed shortly thereafter by PDGF-like material in the culture media. In addition, the TGFβ1 treated cells underwent DNA synthesis with delayed kinetics relative to direct PDGF stimulation. It was recently demonstrated that in human skin fibroblasts, TGFβ can also stimulate autocrine production of PDGF-like peptides [44]. Taken together, these data suggest that the mitogenic effect of TGFβ on mouse embryo fibroblasts may be by the induction of PDGF-like molecules which can then act in an autocrine fashion on these cells. Of interest are the recent reports that a maternally-encoded PDGF mRNA is found in *Xenopus* embryos [45]. It should also be noted that most epithelial cell types, which are not stimulated by TGFβ, lack PDGF receptors.

In contrast to their mitogenic effects in some mesenchymal cell types, TGFβ1 and TGFβ2 are highly inhibitory to proliferation in most epithelial cell types as well as others such as some fibroblast cells, endothelial cells, lymphoid cells, and myeloid cells [46, 47]. Using the BALB/MK mouse keratinocyte cell line as a model system for TGFβ effects on epithelial cells, our lab has shown that picomolar concentrations of TGFβ1, TGFβ2, and TGFβ3 can reversibly inhibit the growth of these keratinocytes in monolayer (for a more comprehensive review of TGFβ effects on keratinocytes see [48] or [49]). In addition to their in vitro effects, in vivo studies of liver regeneration in the rat following partial hepatectomy demonstrate that nanomolar concentrations of TGFβ1 or TGFβ2 can inhibit the early proliferative phase of regeneration [50] and may regulate in vivo liver growth [51]. Likewise, in vivo studies of mouse mammary growth have revealed that TGFβ1 can reversibly inhibit the proliferation of mammary duct epithelium [52, 53].

While the proliferation of most normal epithelial cell lines is greatly inhibited by TGFβ1, several neoplastic cell lines are unaffected by the addition of TGFβ1. It has been widely hypothesized that by escaping the negative regulatory effects of the TGFβs, through loss of the receptor, loss of the post-receptor signal, loss of latent-form activation, loss of TGFβ synthesis capability, etc., some cells may lose their ability to regulate their growth and therefore form tumors. For example, radioreceptor assays indicate that the squamous carcinoma cell line SCC-25 may have lost the ability to bind TGFβ1 [54]. Likewise, the human A549 lung carcinoma cell line is unable to activate the latent form of TGFβ1 [55]. MCF-7 cells, derived from a human breast cancer, are inhibited by both TGFβ1 as well as TGFβ2 and exhibit reduced synthesis of TGFβ1 when stimulated to grow with β-estradiol [56, 57].

The mechanism of TGFβ inhibition of epithelial cells remains enigmatic. Using the BALB/MK system, Coffey et al. have demonstrated that TGFβ1 can inhibit the stimulation of keratinocytes by epidermal growth factor (EGF) [58]. The TGFβ1 treatment did not affect the ligand-receptor interactions of EGF, nor did it effect the EGF induction of c-*fos*. However, TGFβ1 did selectively suppress EGF induction of c-*myc* expression and DNA synthesis. Hence, in light of reports implicating c-*myc* as playing a causal role in cell proliferation, it has been postulated that the inhibitory actions of TGFβ may be through selective suppression of genes such as c-*myc*.

TGFβ Effects on Extracellular Matrix

The role of the extracellular matrix (ECM) during embryonic development is primarily one of tissue modeling. The ECM not only provides a scaffolding for organogenesis, it also functions in the stabilization of proteins and polysaccharides that are important in the proliferation and differentiation of embryonic tissues [59]. TGFβ1 has been shown to have profound effects on the ECM. The modulation of the ECM by TGFβ1 is bipartite; TGFβ1 not only stimulates the expression of matrix components which give rise to the ECM [60–64], it also inhibits the formation of proteases which will degrade the ECM by 1) decreasing protease expression and 2) increasing the expression of protease inhibitors. Early studies of the effects of TGFβ treatment of embryonic fibroblasts showed that TGFβ1 increases the production of fibronectin and type I collagen [65–67] apparently through an increase in transcription rate as well as an increase in message stability for these proteins. TGFβ1 also increases the expression of the integrins in fibroblast cells. In contrast to its effects on most mesenchymal cells, TGFβ1 has been reported to inhibit proliferation of palatal mesenchymal cells and to decrease their ability to produce ECM components. Thus TGFβ1 is thought to play some role in palate formation [68].

One of the early effects of TGFβ1 on embryonic lung fibroblasts is the stimulation of plasminogen activator inhibitor-1 (PAI-1) [69–71]. TGFβ1 causes an overall 50-fold enhancement of PAI-1 message over a period of 8 h. Concomitant with the increase in PAI-1 message, TGFβ1 decreases plasminogen activator (PA) activity; (both urokinase-type PA and tissue-type PA) [72]. In addition, TGFβ1 has also been shown to increase the expression of the metalloprotease inhibitor TIMP [73], to decrease the expression of the proteases, collagenase and stromelysin [74], and to act as a chemotactic factor for fibroblasts [75] perhaps thereby contributing to the stimulation of connective tissue formation [76]. Interestingly, transcripts for both TIMP and the metalloproteases stromelysin and collagenase have been localized in the deciduum as well as in the pre-implantation embryo suggesting that these proteins may play a role during early development [77, 78]. Hence, the regulation of these molecules by TGFβ1 may modulate processes involved in implantation [79]. Proteases are also thought to be involved in neoplastic events, especially metastasis [80, 81].

Considering the significance of the ECM in tissue modelling during embryonic development, its modulation by TGFβ1 would appear to be one of the primary functions of this molecule in embryogenesis. In light of the proposed role of PA in embryonic tissue remodelling, the regulation of this molecule by TGFβ1 may be especially important [82].

TGFβ Effects on Cell Differentiation

One of the most important processes occuring during development is the differentiation of an uncommitted 'primitive' cell into a cell which has specialized functions. Data indicate that TGFβ1 may play a role in the regulation of differentiation in several cell types.

TGFβ1 has been reported to modulate expression of the differentiated phenotype in various cell types of mesenchymal origin. Using a mouse 3T3-11 preadipocyte model system, it was found that picomolar concentrations of TGFβ1 could prevent the conversion of these cells to fully differentiated adipocytes [83, 84]. TGFβ1 was found to bind to high affinity receptors on these cells and to inhibit all morphological conversion without inhibiting mitosis. In addition to the inhibition of adipocyte differentiation, TGFβ1 has been shown to suppress myogenic differentiation as well [85–89]. Using embryonic cell lines from chick, quail, rat and mouse, TGFβ1 at a concentration of 10–20 picomolar has been shown to reversibly inhibit the morphological conversion of undifferentiated myoblasts. TGFβ1 was found to be non-mitogenic for these cells, suggesting that the inhibition was not dependent on cell proliferation.

While TGFβ1 inhibits differentiation of pre-adipocytes and pre-myocytes, it appears to potently stimulate expression of the differentiated phenotype in some other mesenchymally-derived cell types. TGFβ1 and TGFβ2 have been shown to induce rat muscle mesenchymal (RMM) cells to differentiate into cartilage-type cells [90-92]. Treatment of RMM cells with TGFβ1 prompts these cells to assume a cartilage-type morphology and to synthesize the cartilage-specific proteins, cartilage proteoglycan and type II collagen. This induction takes place in the absence of DNA synthesis. In contrast to its effects on chondrogenesis [93], TGFβ1 does not appear to stimulate differentiation of osteoblasts. Interestingly however, TGFβ1 is a potent regulator of osteoblasts and cells treated with TGFβ1 show a range of effects (for a review see [94]). For example, TGFβ1 can either stimulate or inhibit proliferation, increase the expression of osteonectin, osteopontin, and collagen, or decrease osteocalcin expression [95-100]. TGFβ1 and TGFβ2 can also induce in vivo bone formation [101]. It was found that osteoblasts can produce TGFβ1 at approximately 200 ng/g of wet tissue. Although this is roughly half of the amount found in platelets, bone is the tissue with the greatest amount of TGFβ1. Hence, TGFβ1 produced by osteoblasts may act upon neighboring cell types such as chondroblasts and fibroblasts and may be involved in processes such as bone resorption, all of which may be important to bone formation.

The role of TGFβ in epithelial cell differentiation is not as clear as for the mesenchymal cells. TGFβ1 has been reported to cause both human bronchial epithelial cells [102] and rabbit tracheal epithelial cells [103] to undergo squamous differentiation; however, this may simply be due to the inhibition of proliferation by TGFβ1. Studies have also suggested that TGFβ1 can cause terminal differentiation in rat intestinal crypt epithelial (IEC-6) cells [104] but other investigators have been unable to repeat this work [105]. Recent studies indicate that TGFβ1 is able to inhibit the differentiation of adrenocortical cells [106] and precursor lymphocytes [107]. In the embryonic heart, TGFβ1 has been reported to mediate the transformation of endothelial cells into mesenchymal progenitor cells of the valves and membranous septa [108]. However, TGFβ1 does not alter differentiation during the process of inhibiting proliferation of skin keratinocytes [58].

TGFβ Effects on Mesoderm Induction

The body plan and pattern of future organ anlagen are determined through inductive events very early in development. In vertebrate development, the initial patterning event is the induction of mesoderm and its subsequent elaboration of secondary inductive processes. Although the induction of mesoderm is thought to occur in all vertebrates, most studies of this process have used amphibian embryos due to the ease with which they can be viewed and manipulated. While several members of the TGFβ family have been implicated as playing some role in mesoderm induction, it is by no means clear what that role is. However, due to the pioneering work of Smith [109, 110] and Melton [111], a more lucid picture is starting to emerge (for a comprehensive review of mesoderm induction see [112]).

The reports concerning the ability of TGFβ1 to induce mesoderm formation are contradictory. Studies using early gastrulae of *Triturus alpestris* suggest that purified human TGFβ1 can direct differentiation of isolated ectoderm tissue into mesoderm [113]. However, this occurs in only 61 % of the explants and at relatively high concentrations of TGFβ1. In contrast to this data, other investigators have reported that experiments with tissue derived from *Xenopus laevis* blastulae indicate that TGFβ1 alone is unable to induce mesoderm formation from isolated ectodermal explants [114, 115]. However, when these explants are treated with a combination of TGFβ1 and basic FGF (bFGF), these proteins are able to act synergistically to induce cardiac actin expression, a marker for mesoderm [115]. To further complicate this matter, another group of investigators has reported that at no concentration of TGFβ1, with or without bFGF, was mesoderm formation in ectodermal explants obtained [116]. However, a strong induction of cardiac actin expression was obtained when the explants were treated with TGFβ2 alone. Addition of bFGF had little or no synergistic effect. Furthermore, it was found that antibodies directed against TGFβ2 but not against TGFβ1 could block the inductive effect of another mesoderm-inducer, XTC-MIF [116]. To date, neither a *Xenopus* TGFβ2 homolog nor any effects of exogenous TGFβ3 on mesoderm expression have been reported. Therefore, while it is unclear what role TGFβ1, TGFβ2 and TGFβ3 may play in vertebrate mesoderm induction, it appears that the endogenous inducing molecule is most likely a member of the TGFβ family.

XTC-MIF, derived from the conditioned medium of the *Xenopus* XTC cell line, is a remarkably potent inducer of mesoderm formation [109, 110]. Evidence suggests that XTC-MIF is a member of the TGFβ family [116], however, as yet no sequence information for this molecule has been reported and therefore no definitive evidence for transcripts or protein has yet been detected in the embryo. Nonetheless, due to its powerful mesoderm inducing ability and its isolation from a *Xenopus* cell line, XTC-MIF must be considered as a candidate endogenous mesoderm-inducing molecule in the *Xenopus* embryo [112].

Another possible endogenous inducer of mesoderm is the protein product of the *Xenopus* Vg-1 gene, a member of the distantly-related group of the TGFβ family [20, 117–120]. Vg-1 comprises 0.05–0.1% of the total poly(A)$^+$RNA pool in the oocyte and in situ hybridization reveals that in the early unfertilized oocyte, Vg-1 transcripts can be located throughout the egg. However, as oogenesis proceeds, the Vg-1 transcripts begin to localize to the vegetal (presumptive endoderm) half of the egg and following fertilization, the Vg-1 message appears to move toward the animal (presumptive ecto-derm) pole. This is approximately the pattern one would expect of an endo-genous mesoderm inducer. Still, however compelling this indirect evidence may be, at present Vg-1 has not yet been shown to induce mesoderm forma-tion. Interestingly, Lyons et al. have demonstrated that mRNA for Vgr-1, a gene cloned from an 8.5 day post coitum mouse cDNA library [21], can be localized in both fertilized and unfertilized murine oocytes [121]. Vgr-1 is another member of the distantly-related group of the TGFβ family.

TGFβ Embryonic Expression

In the foregoing discussion it has been demonstrated that members of the TGFβ family have profound and unique effects on embryonic cells of varied origins thereby implicating these family members in developmen-tally important events. Strong evidence to support this comes from studies which have localized mRNA and protein of the various TGFβ family mem-bers to unique sites in the embryo consistent with many of the in vitro studies done with these family members.

Using the technique of in situ hybridization, several different groups have demonstrated the presence of TGFβ1 mRNA in human as well as murine embryonic tissues [122–125]. The most extensive of these studies, by Lehnert et al., showed TGFβ1 mRNA to be expressed at high levels in hepatic megakaryocytes and bone as well as several epithelially derived tis-sues such as thymus, thyroid, whisker follicles, tooth bud, submandibular gland, and the endocardial portion of the developing heart valves [122]. Another group, using immunohistochemical staining, has demonstrated the expression of TGFβ1 protein in many different organs in late stage mouse development; however, questions concerning the specificity of the polyclonal antibodies used in these studies remain [126].

Like TGFβ1, TGFβ2 mRNA has also been localized in the embryo. In situ hybridization studies have revealed that TGFβ2 transcripts can be found in a variety of tissues including bone, cartilage, tendon, gut, blood vessels, skin and fetal placenta [127]. The TGFβ2 message is generally found in the mesenchymal component of these tissues in areas adjacent to an overlying epithelium, however, some areas of epithelial expression are observed. The pattern of TGFβ2 expression in these tissues appears to be consistent with a role for this molecule in mesenchymal-epithelial interactions and tissue morphogenesis. Reports of TGFβ2 mRNA expression as revealed by Northern blot hybridization analysis support the in situ data [128].

Northern blot hybridization data has revealed that similar to TGFβ1 and TGFβ2, TGFβ3 mRNA can be detected in the developing mouse embryo [129]. TGFβ3 transcripts can be seen as early as 10.5 days post coitum and relative levels of TGFβ3 message appear to increase as development proceeds. Interestingly, in situ hybridization data demonstrate that TGFβ3 appears to localize to many of the same embryonic tissues and cell types as TGFβ1 and TGFβ2 and at the same times of development [130, 131]. Nonetheless, differences in expression do exist. In addition, avian TGFβ3 and TGFβ4 have been cloned from an embryonic chicken chondrocyte library suggesting that these molecules may also play some role in chicken chondrogenesis [13, 132].

Recent studies have now revealed that in addition to its expression in the oocyte, Vgr-1 mRNA is also expressed in a number of tissues throughout murine embryogenesis [121]. High levels of Vgr-1 message are seen in late stage embryos in the suprabasal layers of the skin, cervix, vagina, and esophagus. Transcripts are also seen in the hypertrophic cartilage of the developing bone. In addition to the Vgr-1 mRNA expression, these studies demonstrated the localization of BMP-2a mRNA expression in several embryonic tissues in temporally and spatially distinct patterns from those seen for Vgr-1, TGFβ1 and TGFβ2 [121]. BMP-2a is a member of the distantly-related group of the TGFβ family.

Conclusion

The available evidence clearly suggests that members of both the closely-related and distantly-related groups of the TGFβ family are involved in embryonic events. Just exactly what the role(s) is/are, however, remains to be strictly defined. Nevertheless, the present studies have thus far raised several fundamental questions concerning the role of growth factors during vertebrate development. For example, TGFβ1, TGFβ2 and TGFβ3, molecules which show very similar activities in most in vitro assays, are all expressed in many of the same tissues and at the same time during development; what is the purpose of this apparent redundancy? One might postulate that these molecules have subtle yet significant differences in biological activity which may not be seen in many of the tissue culture assays used to characterize proteins. Alternatively, these differences may be manifest only in certain situations such as those which may occur during development. Indeed, it has been widely hypothesized that these molecules may play very different roles in the embryo and adult; hence, those in vitro assays which use non-embryonic cell types may not reveal the subtle differences which exist. Lastly, the local environment and general protein milieu may have profound effects that cannot be duplicated in the culture dish. Hopefully, further studies will reveal the true function(s) of these molecules in normal embryonic development and perhaps provide clues as to what role they may play in neoplasia.

References

1   Adamson ED: Oncogenes in development. Development 1987; 99:449–471.
2   Weinberg RA: Oncogenes, antioncogenes and the molecular basis of multistep carcinogenesis. Cancer Res 1989;49:3713–3721.
3   Moses HL, Branum EB, Proper JA, et al: Transforming growth factor production by chemically transformed cells. Cancer Res 1981;41:2842–2848.
4   Roberts AB, Anzano MA, Lamb LC, et al: New class of transforming growth factors potentiated by epidermal growth factor: isolation from non-neoplastic tissues. Proc Natl Acad Sci USA 1981;78:5339–5343.
5   Massagué J: The TGF-β family of growth and differentiation factors. Cell 1987; 49:437–438.
6   Derynck R, Lindquist PB, Lee A, et al: A new type of transforming growth factor-β, TGF-β3. EMBO J 1988;7:3737–3743.
7   Gentry L, Lioubin MN, Purchio AF, et al: Molecular events in the processing of recombinant type 1 pre-pro-transforming growth factor β to mature polypeptide. Mol Cell Biol 1988;8:4162–4168.
8   Lyons RM, Keski-Oja J, Moses HL: Proteolytic activation of latent transforming factor-β from fibroblast conditioned medium. J Cell Biol 1988;106:1659–1665.
9   Lyons RM, Gentry LE, Purchio AF, et al: Mechanism of activation of latent recombinant transforming growth factor β1 by plasmin. J Cell Biol 1990;110:1361–1367.
10   Derynck R, Jarret JA, Chen EY, et al: Human transforming growth factor-β complementary DNA sequence and expression in normal and transformed cells. Nature 1985;315:701–705.

11   Madisen L, Webb NR, Rose TM, et al: Transforming growth factor-$\beta 2$: cDNA cloning and sequence analysis. DNA 1988;7:1–8.

12   ten Dijke P, Hansen P, Iwata KK, et al: Identification of another member of the transforming growth factor type β gene family. Proc Natl Acad Sci USA 1988;85:4715–4719.

13   Jakowlew SB, Dillard P, Sporn MB, et al: Complementary deoxyribonucleic acid cloning of a messenger ribonucleic acid encoding transforming growth factor $\beta 4$ from chicken embryo chondrocytes. Mol Endo 1988;2:1186–1195.

14   Sporn MB, Roberts AB, Wakefield LM, et al: Some recent advances in the chemistry and biology of transforming growth factor-beta. J Cell Biol 1987;105:1039–1045.

15   Sharples K, Plowman GD, Rose TM, et al: Cloning and sequence analysis of simian transforming growth factor-beta cDNA. DNA 1987;6:239–244.

16   Derynck R, Jarret JA, Chen EY, et al: The murine transforming growth factor-β precursor. J Biol Chem 1986;261:4377–4379.

17   Cate RL, Mattaliano RJ, Hession C, et al: Isolation of the bovine and human genes for Müllerian inhibiting substance and expression of the human gene in animal cells. Cell 1986;45:685–698.

18   Mason AJ, Hayflick JS, Ling NL, et al: Complementary DNA sequences of ovarian follicular fluid inhibin show precursor structure and homology with transforming growth factor-β. Nature 1985;318:659–663.

19   Wozney JM, Rosen V, Celeste AJ, et al: Novel regulators of bone formation: Molecular clones and activities. Science 1988;242:1528–1534.

20   Weeks DL, Melton DA: A maternal mRNA localized to the vegetal hemisphere in *Xenopus* eggs codes for a growth factor related to TGF-β. Cell 1987;51:861–867.

21   Lyons K, Graycar JL, Lee A, et al: Vgr-1, a mammalian gene related to *Xenopus vg-1* and a new member of the TGFβ gene superfamily. Proc Natl Acad Sci USA 1989; 86:4554–4558.

22   Padgett RW, St Johnson RD, Gelbart WM: A transcript from a *Drosophila* pattern gene predicts a protein homologous to the transforming growth factor-β gene family. Nature 1987;325:81–84.

23   Segarini PR, Rosen DM, Seyedin SM: Binding of transforming growth factor-beta to cell surface proteins varies with cell type. Mol Endo 1989;3:261–272.

24   Frolik CA, Wakefield LM, Smith DM, et al: Characterization of a membrane receptor for transforming growth factor-β in normal rat kidney fibroblasts. J Biol Chem 1984;259:10995–11000.

25   Massagué J, Like B: Cellular receptors for type β transforming growth factor. Ligand binding and affinity labeling in human and rodent lines. J Biol Chem 1985; 260:2636–2645.

26   Tucker RF, Branum EL, Shipley GD, et al: Specific binding to cultured cells of 125I-labeled transforming growth factor-type β from human platelets. Proc Natl Acad Sci USA 1984;8:6757–6761.

27   Cheifetz S, Like B, Massagué J: Cellular distribution of type I and type II receptors for transforming growth factor β. J Biol Chem 1986;261:9972–9978.

28   Massagué J: Subunit structure of a high affinity receptor for type β transforming growth factor. Evidence for a disulfide linked glycosylated receptor complex. J Biol Chem 1986;260:7059–7066.

29   Massagué J, Cheifetz S, Ignotz R: TGF-β receptors and actions. J Cell Biol 1988;106-(suppl 12A):181.

30   Cheifetz S, Weatherbee JA, Tsang ML-S, et al: The transforming growth factor-beta system, a complex pattern of cross-reactive ligands and receptors. Cell 1987;48:409–415.

31   Boyd FT, Massagué J: Transforming growth factor-beta inhibition of epithelial cell proliferation linked to the expression of a 53-kDa membrane receptor. J Biol Chem 1989;264:2272–2278.

32   Libby J, Mortinez R, Weber MJ: Tyrosine phosphorylation in cells treated with transforming growth factor-beta. J Cell Physiol 1986;129:159–166.

33   Fine LG, Holley RW, Nasri H, et al: BSC-1 growth inhibitor transforms a mitogenic stimulus into a hypertrophic stimulus for renal proximal tubular cells: Relationship to Na^+/H^+ antiport activity. Proc Natl Acad Sci USA 1985;82:6163–6166.

34   Murthy US, Anzano MA, Stadel JM, et al: Coupling of TGF-beta-induced mitogenesis to G-protein activation in AKR-2B cells. Biochem Biophys Res Comm 1988; 152:1228–1235.

35   Howe PH, Bascom CC, Cunningham MR, et al: Multiple transducing pathways regulate TGFβ1 action: Evidence for both G protein dependent and independent signaling. Cancer Res 1989;49:6024–6031.

36   Howe PH, Leof EB: Transforming growth factor β1 treatment of AKR-2B cells is coupled through a pertussis-toxin-sensitive G-protein(s). Biochem J 1989;261:879–886.

37   Rizzino A: Appearance of high affinity receptors for type β transforming growth factor during differentiation of murine embryonal carcinoma cells. Cancer Res 1987; 47:4386–4390.

38   Rollins BJ, O'Connell TM, Bennett G, et al: Environment-dependent growth inhibition of human epidermal keratinocytes by recombinant human transforming growth factor beta. J Cell Physiol 139:455–462.

39   Moses HL, Tucker RF, Leof EB, et al: Type β transforming growth factor is a growth stimulator and a growth inhibitor, in Feramisco J, Ozanne B, Stiles B (eds): Growth factors and transformation. Cancer cells 3. Cold Spring Harbor, NY, Cold Spring Harbor Press, 1985, pp 54–71.

40   Centrella M, McCarthy TL, Canalis E: Transforming growth factor beta is a bifunctional regulator of replication and collagen synthesis in osteoblast-enriched cell cultures from fetal rat bone. J Biol Chem 1987;262:2869–2874.

41   Robey PG, Young MF, Flanders KC: Osteoblasts synthesize and respond to TGF-beta in vitro. J Cell Biol 1987;105:457–463.

42   Graycar JL, Miller DA, Arrick BA, et al: Human transforming growth factor-β3: recombinant expression, purification and biological activities in comparison with transforming growth factors-β1 and β2. Mol Endo 1989;3:1977–1986.

43   Leof EB, Proper JA, Goustin AS, et al: Induction of c-sis mRNA and activity similar to platelet-derived growth factor by transforming growth factor β: A proposed model for indirect mitogenesis involving autocrine activity. Proc Natl Acad Sci USA 1986; 83:2453–2457.

44   Soma Y, Grotendorst GR: TGF-beta stimulates primary human fibroblast DNA synthesis via an autocrine production of PDGF-related peptides. J Cell Physiol 1989; 140:246–253.

45   Mercola M, Melton DA, Stiles CD: Platelet-derived growth factor A chain is mater-
      nally encoded in *Xenopus* embryos. Science 1989;241:1223–1225.
46   Tucker RF, Shipley GD, Moses HL, et al: Growth inhibitor from BSC-1 cells closely
      related to type beta TGF. Science 1984; 226:705–707.
47   Moses HL, Leof EB: Transforming growth factor-β, in Kahn P, Graf T (eds): Oncoge-
      nes and growth control. Heidelberg, Springer, 1986, pp 51–57.
48   Bascom CC, Sipes NJ, Coffey RJ, et al: Regulation of epithelial cell proliferation by
      transforming growth factors. J Cell Biochem 1989;39:25–32.
49   Barnard JA, Bascom CC, Lyons RM, et al: Transforming growth factor beta in the
      control of epidermal proliferation. Am J Med Sci 1988;31:159–163.
50   Russell WE, Coffey RJ, Ouelette AJ, et al: Type β transforming growth factor revers-
      ibly inhibits the early proliferative response to partial hepatectomy in the rat. Proc
      Natl Acad Sci USA 1988;85:5126–5130.
51   Braun L, Mead JE, Panzica M, et al: Transforming growth factor beta mRNA increa-
      ses during liver regeneration: a possible paracrine mechanism of growth regulation.
      Proc Natl Acad Sci USA 1988;85:1539–1543.
52   Daniel CW, Silberstein GB, Van Horn K, et al: TGFβ1-induced inhibition of mouse
      mammary ductal growth: Developmental specificity and characterization. Dev Biol
      1989;135:20–30.
53   Silberstein GB, Daniel CW: Reversible inhibition of mammary gland growth by
      transforming growth factor-beta. Science 1987;237:291–293.
54   Shipley GD, Pittelkow MR, Wille JJ, et al: Reversible inhibition of normal human
      prokeratinocyte proliferation by type β transforming growth factor-growth inhibitor
      in serum-free medium. Cancer Res 1986;46:2068–2071.
55   Wakefield LM, Smith DM, Masui T, et al: Distribution and modulation of the cellular
      receptor for transfoming growth factor beta. J Cell Biol 1987;105:965–975.
56   Zugmaier G, Ennis BW, Deschauer B, et al: Transforming growth factors type β1 and
      β2 are equipotent growth inhibitors of human breast cancer cell lines. J Cell Physiol
      1989;141:353–361.
57   Knabbe C, Lippman ME, Wakefield LM, et al: Evidence that transforming growth
      factor β is a hormonally regulated negative growth factor in human breast cancer
      cells. Cell 1987;48:417–428.
58   Coffey RJ Jr., Sipes NJ, Bascom CC, et al: Growth modulation of mouse keratino-
      cytes by transforming growth factors. Cancer Res 1988;48:1596–1602.
59   Hay ED: Collagen and embryonic development in Hay ED (ed): Cell Biology of
      Extracellular Matrix. New York, Plenum Publishing 1981, vol 3, pp 65–71.
60   Yoshida K, Yokozaki H, Niimoto M, et al: Expression of TGF-beta and procollagen
      type I and type III in human gastric carcinomas. Int J Cancer 1989;44:394–398.
61   Balza E, Borsi L, Allemanni G, et al: Transforming growth factor beta regulates the
      levels of different fibronectin isoforms in normal human cultured fibroblasts. FEBS
      Lett 1988;228:42–44.
62   Bassols A, Massagué J: Transforming growth factor beta regulates the expression and
      strucutre of extracellular matrix chondroitin/dermatan sulfate proteoglycans. J Biol
      Chem 1988;263:3039–3045.
63   Inoue H, Kato Y, Iwamoto M, et al: Stimulation of cartilage-matrix proteoglycan synth-
      esis by morphologically transformed chondrocytes grown in the presence of fibroblast
      growth factor and transforming growth factor-beta. J Cell Physiol 1989; 138:329–337.

64　Ignotz RA, Massagué J: Transforming growth factor-β stimulates the expression of fibronectin and collagen and their incorporation into the extracellular matrix. J Biol Chem 1986;261:4337–4345.

65　Ignotz RA, Endo R, Massagué J: Regulation of fibronectin and type I collagen mRNA levels by transforming growth factor-β. J Biol Chem 1987;262:6443–6446.

66　Raghow R, Postlethwaite AE, Keski-Oja J, et al: Transforming growth factor β increases steady state levels of type I procollagen and fibronectin messenger RNAs posttranscriptionally in cultured human dermal fibroblasts. J Clin Invest 1987;79:1285–1288.

67　Blatti SP, Foster DN, Moses HL, et al: Induction of fibronectin messenger RNA is a primary response to epidermal growth factor stimulation of AKR-2B cells. Proc Nat Acad Sci USA 1988;85:1119–1123.

68　Ferguson MWJ: Palate development: Mechanisms and malformations. Irish J Med Sci 1987;156:309–315.

69　Laiho M, Saksela O, Andreasen PA, et al: Enhanced production and extracellular deposition of the endothelial-type plasminogen activator inhibitor in cultured human lung fibroblasts by transforming growth factor-β. J Cell Biol 1986;103:2403–2410.

70　Lund LR, Riccio A, Andreasen PA, et al: Transforming growth factor-beta is a strong and fast acting positive regulator of the level of type-1 plasminogen activator inhibitor mRNA in WI-38 human lung fibroblasts. EMBO J 1987;6:1281–1286.

71　Keski-Oja J, Raghow R, Sawdey M, et al: Regulation of mRNAs for type-1 plasminogen activator inhibitor, fibronectin and type I procollagen by transforming growth factor-beta, divergent responses in lung fibroblasts and carcinoma cells. J Biol Chem 1988;263:3111–3115.

72　Keski-Oja J, Blasi F, Leof EB, et al: Regulation of the synthesis and activity of urokinase plasminogen activator in human lung carcinoma cells by transforming growth factor-β. J Cell Biol 1988;106:451–459.

73　Edwards DR, Murphy G, Reynold JJ, et al: Transforming growth factor beta modulates the expression of collagenase and metalloproteinase inhibitor. EMBO J 1987; 6:1899–1904.

74　Matrisian LM, Leroy P, Ruhlmann C, et al: Isolation of the oncogene and growth factor-induced transin gene: complex control in rat fibroblasts. Mol Cell Biol 1986; 6:1679–1686.

75　Postlethwaite AE, Keski-Oja J, Moses HL, et al: Stimulation of the chemotactic migration of human fibroblasts by transforming growth factor β. J Exp Med 1987;165:251–256.

76　Roberts AB, Sporn MB, Assoian RK, et al: Transforming growth factor type β: Rapid induction of fibrosis and angiogenesis in vivo and stimulation of collagen formation in vitro. Proc Natl Acad Sci USA 1986;83:4167–4171.

77　Nomura S, Hogan BLM, Willis AJ, et al: Developmental expression of tissue inhibitor of metalloproteinase (TIMP) RNA. Development 1989;105:575–583.

78　Brenner CA, Adler RR, Rappolee DA, et al: Genes for extracellular matrix-degrading metalloproteinases and their inhibitor, TIMP, are expressed during early mammalian development. Genes Dev 1989;3:848–859.

79　Sappino A-P, Huarte J, Belin D, et al: Plasminogen activators in tissue remodeling and invasion: mRNA localization in mouse ovaries and implanting embryos. J Cell Biol 1989;109:2471–2479.

80   Rifkin DB, Moscatelli D, Gross J, et al: Proteases, angiogenesis, and invasion, in Nicolson GL, Milas L (eds): Cancer Invasion and Metastasis: Biological and Therapeutic Aspects. New York, Raven Press, 1984, pp 187–200.

81   Dano K, Andreasen PA, Grondahl-Hansen J, et al: Plasminogen activators, tissue degradation and cancer. Adv Cancer Res 1985;44:139–266.

82   Strickland S, Reich E, Sherman M: Plasminogen activator in early embryogenesis: enzyme production by trophoblasts and parietal endoderm. Cell 1976;9:231–240.

83   Ignotz RA, Massagué J: Type beta transforming growth factor controls the adipogenic differentiation of 3T3 fibroblasts. Proc Natl Acad Sci USA 1985;82:8530–8534.

84   Torti FM, Torti SV, Larrick JW, et al: Modulation of adipocyte differentiation by tumor necrosis factor and transforming growth factor beta. J Cell Biol 1989; 108:1105–1113.

85   Massagué J, Cheifetz S, Endo T, et al: Type beta transforming growth factor is an inhibitor of myogenic differentiation. Proc Natl Acad Sci USA 1986;83:8206–8210.

86   Olson EN, Sternberg E, Hu JS, et al: Regulation of myogenic differentiation by type beta transforming growth factor. J Cell Biol 1986;103:1799–1805.

87   Florini JR, Roberts AB, Ewton DZ, et al: Transforming growth factor-beta: A very potent inhibitor of myoblast differentiation, identical to the differentiation inhibitor secreted by Buffalo rat liver cells. J Biol Chem 1986;261:16509–16513.

88   Ewton DZ, Spizz G, Olson EN, et al: Decrease in transforming growth factor-beta binding and action during differentiation in muscle cells. J Biol Chem 1988; 263:4029–4032.

89   Florini JR, Magri KA: Effects of growth factors on myogenic differentiation. Am J Physiol 1989;256:701–711.

90   Seyedin SM, Thomas TC, Thompson AY, et al: Purification and characterization of two cartilage-inducing factors from bovine demineralized bone. Proc. Natl Sci USA 1985;82:2267–2271.

91   Seyedin SM, Thompson AY, Bentz H, et al: Cartilage-inducing factor-A: Apparent identity to transforming growth factor-beta. J Biol Chem 1986;261:5692–5695.

92   Seyedin SM, Segarini PR, Rosen DM, et al: Cartilage-inducing factor-B is a unique protein structurally and functionally related to transforming growth factor-beta. J Biol Chem 1987;262:1946–1949.

93   Kulyk WM, Rodgers BJ, Greer K, et al: Promotion of embryonic chick limb cartilage differentiation by transforming growth factor-β. Dev Biol 1989;135:424–430.

94   Centrella M, McCarthy TL, Canalis E: Skeletal tissue and transforming growth factor beta. FASEB J 1988;2:3066–3073.

95   Centrella M, McCarthy TL, Canalis E: Transforming growth factor beta is a bifunctional regulator of replication and collagen synthesis in osteoblast-enriched cell cultures from fetal rat bone. J Biol Chem 1987;262:2869–2874.

96   Centrella M, McCarthy TL, Cannalis E: Mitogenesis in fetal rat bone cells simultaneously exposed to type beta transforming growth factor and other growth regulators. FASEB J 1987;1:312–317.

97   Noda M, Rodan GA: Type beta transforming growth factor (TGFbeta) regulation of alkaline phosphatase expression and other phenotype-related mRNAs in osteoblastic rat osteosarcoma cells. J Cell Physiol 1987;133:426–437.

98   Globus RK, Patterson-Buckendahl P, Gospodarowicz D: Regulation of bovine bone
      cell proliferation by fibroblast growth factor and transforming growth factor beta.
      Endocrinology 1988;123:98–105.
99   Pfeilschifter J, DSouza SM, Mundy GR: Effects of transforming growth factor-beta
      on osteoblastic osteosarcoma cells. Endocrinology 1987;121:212–218.
100   Noda M: Transcriptional regulation of osteocalcin production by transforming
      growth factor-beta in rat osteoblast-like cells. Endocrinology 1989;124:612–617.
101   Noda M, Camilliere JJ: In vivo stimulation of bone formation by transforming
      growth factor-beta. Endocrinology 1989;124:2991–2994.
102   Masui T, Wakefield LM, Lechner JF, et al: Type beta transforming growth factor is
      the primary differentiation-inducing serum factor for normal human bronchial epi-
      thelial cells. Proc Natl Acad Sci USA 1986;83:2438–2442.
103   Jetten AM, Shirley JE, Stoner G: Regulation of proliferation and differentiation of
      respiratory tract epithelial cells by TGF-beta. Exp Cell Res 1986;167:539–549.
104   Kurokowa M, Lynch K, Podolsky DK: Effects of growth factors on an intestinal epi-
      thelial cell line: Transforming growth factor beta inhibits proliferation and stimulates
      differentiation. Biochem Biophys Res Comm 1987;142:775–782.
105   Barnard JA, Beauchamp RD, Coffey RJ, et al: Regulation of intestinal epithelial cell
      growth by transforming growth factor type β. Proc Natl Acad Sci USA 1989;86:1578–1582.
106   Riopel L, Branchaud CL, Goodyer CG, et al: Growth-inhibitory effect of TGF-beta
      on human fetal adrenal cells in primary monolayer culture. J Cell Physiol 1989;
      140:233–238.
107   Jin B, Scott JL, Vadas MA, et al: TGF beta down-regulates TLiSA1 expression and
      inhibits the differentiation of precursor lymphocytes into CTL and LAK cells. Immu-
      nology 1989;66:570–576.
108   Potts JD, Runyan RB: Epithelial-mesenchymal cell transformation in the embryonic
      heart can be mediated, in part, by transforming growth factor β. Dev Biol 1989;
      134:392–401.
109   Smith JC: A mesoderm inducing factor is produced by a *Xenopus* cell line. Develop-
      ment 1987;99:3–14.
110   Smith JC, Yaqoob M, Symes K: Purification, partial characterization and biological
      properties of the XTC mesoderm-inducing factor. Development 1988;103:591–600.
111   Altaba AR, Melton DA: Interaction between growth factors and homeobox genes in
      the establishment of anterior-posterior polarity in frog embryos. Nature 1989;
      341:33–38.
112   Smith JC: Mesoderm induction and mesoderm-inducing factors in early amphibian
      development. Development 1989;105:665–677.
113   Knöchel W, Born J, Hoppe P, et al: Mesoderm-inducing factors. Naturwissenschaf-
      ten 1987;74:604–606.
114   Slack JMW, Darlington BG, Heath JK, et al: Mesoderm induction in early *Xenopus*
      embryos by heparin-binding growth factors. Nature 1987;326:197–200.
115   Kimelman D, Kirschner M: Synergistic induction of mesoderm by FGF and TGF-
      beta and the identification of an mRNA coding for FGF in the early *Xenopus* embryo.
      Cell 1987;51:869–877.
116   Rosa F, Roberts AB, Danielpour D, et al: Mesoderm induction in amphibians: the
      role of TGF-beta2-like factors. Science 1988;239:783–785.

117 Rebagliati MR, Weeks DL, Harvey RP, et al: Identification and cloning of localized maternal RNA's from *Xenopus* eggs. Cell 1985;42:769–777.

118 Melton DA: Translocation of a localized maternal mRNA to the vegetal pole of *Xenopus* oocytes. Nature 1987;328:80–82.

119 Yisraeli JK, Melton DA: The maternal mRNA Vg1 is correctly localized following injection into *Xenopus* oocytes. Nature 1988;336:592–595.

120 Tannahill D, Melton DA: Localized synthesis of the Vg1 protein during early *Xenopus* development. Development 1989;106:775–785.

121 Lyons KM, Pelton RW, Hogan BLM: Patterns of expression of murine Vgr-1 and BMP-2A RNA suggest that TGFβ-like genes coordinately regulate aspects of embryonic development. Genes Dev 1989;3:1657–1668.

122 Lehnert SA, Akhurst RJ: Embryonic expression pattern of TGF beta type-1 RNA suggests both paracrine and autocrine mechanisms of action. Development 1988; 104:263–273.

123 Sandberg M, Vuorio T, Hirrovan H: Enhanced expression of TGF-β and c-*fos* mRNAs in the growth plates of developing human long bones. Development 1988; 102:461–470.

124 Sandberg M, Autio-Harmainen H, Vuorio E: Localization of the expression of types I, III, and IV collagen, TGF-β1 and c-*fos* genes in developing human calvarial bones. Dev Biol 1988;130:324–334.

125 Wilcox JN, Derynck R: Developmental expression of transforming growth factors alpha and beta in the mouse fetus. Mol Cell Biol 1988;8:3415–3422.

126 Heine UI, Munoz EF, Flanders KC, et al: Role of transforming growth factor-β in the development of the mouse embryo. J Cell Biol 1987;105:2861–2876.

127 Pelton RW, Nomura S, Moses HL, Hogan BLM: Expression of transforming growth factor beta-2 RNA during murine embryogenesis. Development 1989;106:759–767.

128 Miller DA, Lee A, Pelton RW, et al: Murine transforming growth factor-beta2 cDNA sequence and expression in adult tissues and embryos. Mol Endo 1989;3:1108–1114.

129 Miller DA, Lee A, Chen EY, et al: cDNA cloning of the murine TGF-β3 precursor and the comparative expression of the TGF-β1 mRNA in murine embryos and adult tissues. Mol Endo 1989;7:1926–1934.

130 Pelton RW, Hogan BLM, Miller DA, et al: Differential expression of genes encoding TGFs β1, β2 and β3 during murine palate formation. Dev Biol 1990 (in press).

131 Pelton RW, Dickinson ME, Hogan BLM, et al: In situ hybridization analysis of TGF β3 RNA expression during mouse development: Comparative studies with TGF β1 and TGF β2 (submitted).

132 Jakowlew SB, Dillard PJ, Kondaiah P, et al: Complementary deoxyribonucleic acid cloning of a novel transforming growth factor-beta messenger ribonucleic acid from chick embryo chondroyctes. Mol Endo 1988;2:747–755.

R. W. Pelton, Department of Cell Biology, Vanderbilt University Medical School, Nashville, TN, 37232 (USA)

Contrib Oncol, vol 39, pp 115–124 (Karger, Basel, 1990)

Structural and Functional Aspects of Platelet-derived Growth Factor and its Receptors

C.-H. Heldin[a], *B. Westermark*[b]

[a] Ludwig Institute for Cancer Research, Biomedical Center, Uppsala
[b] Department of Pathology, University Hospital, Uppsala, Sweden

The growth of cells is regulated in part by polypeptide factors that stimulate or inhibit cell proliferation (reviewed in [25]). Platelet-derived growth factor (PDGF) is a major growth factor in serum for connective tissue cells (reviewed in [26, 40]). It was originally purified from platelets, and has recently been found to be produced by several different normal cell types (table 1). The sites of production and the target cell specificity of PDGF, suggest a role during embryogenesis, e.g. in the development of the central nervous system and the placenta; in the adult organism PDGF may act as a wound hormone. PDGF may also have an adverse role in pathological situations with increased cell proliferation, such as atherosclerosis, rheumatoid arthritis and fibrosis. In addition, PDGF is frequently produced by malignant cells and may stimulate tumor growth in vivo in autocrine or paracrine manners. The capacity of PDGF to act as an autocrine growth factor was unravelled by the finding that it is similar to the product of the *sis* oncogene of simian sarcoma virus [11, 51]; the transforming properties of this retrovirus was shown to be exerted by a PDGF-like growth factor acting in an autocrine manner (reviewed in [52]). In this communication, we summarize some of the recent advances in our knowledge about PDGF and its mechanism of action.

Different Isoforms of PDGF

PDGF is a dimeric molecule composed of disulphide-bonded A- and B-polypeptide chains. Both chains are synthesized as precursor molecules that undergo proteolytic processing after synthesis and dimerization; in the mature parts of slightly more than 100 amino acids, the two chains are about

Table 1. Normal cell types that produce PDGF*

Cell type	species**	A chain	B chain
Endothelial cells	h, b	+	+
Smooth muscle cells	r	+	
Macrophages	h	+	+
Placental cytotrophoblasts	h		+
Fibroblasts	h	+	
Type-1 astrocytes of the optic nerve	r	+	

* Identified as respector competing activity, immunoprecipitation or mRNA expression. For references see refs. 26, 40

** h, human; r, rat; b, bovine

60 % similar in their amino acid sequence [2]. The A-chain occurs as two variants that differ in the C-terminals due to differential splicing of the gene [4, 39]. Three different isoforms of PDGF have been identified and purified from platelets and transformed cells, -AA, -AB and -BB [20, 27, 48], and are now also available as recombinant proteins [30, 36, 37].

The different isoforms of PDGF show different functional activities on human foreskin fibroblasts; whereas all isoforms induce a mitogenic response, PDGF-AA does not stimulate chemotaxis and actin reorganization [35].

Two Different PDGF Receptor Types

An explanation for the differences in functional activities of the three isoforms of PDGF came through studies of their binding characteristics to cultured cells, which led to the identification of two distinct types of receptors [23, 28]. The α-receptor (also called A-type receptor) binds all isoforms of PDGF with high affinitiy, whereas the β-receptor (also called the B-type receptor) binds PDGF-BB with high affinity, PDGF-AB with lower affinity, and does not bind PDGF-AA with any appreciable affinity. The PDGF α-receptor is synthesized as a precursor of 140 kDa and undergoes maturation to a 170 kDa cell surface expressed receptor [7]. The β-receptor precursor and mature forms are 160 kDa and 180 kDa, respectively [22, 31]. The receptors are turned over fairly rapidly; ligand binding increases the rate of internalization and degradation.

Cloning of cDNA:s for the two PDGF receptors revealed that the predicted protein sequences are very similar [5, 6, 18, 32, 54]. Each receptor has an external part that is composed of five immunoglobulin-like domains and each of the cytoplasmic parts contains a protein tyrosine kinase domain with an inserted sequence without homology to kinase domains. The amino acid similarity is highest, about 80 %, in the kinase domains and in the segment between the plasma membrane and the first part of the kinase domain, and lower, 27–35 %, in the external parts, in the kinase insert domains and in the C-terminal tails. The two PDGF receptors are structurally similar to the receptor for CSF-1 [10] and the c-*kit* product, a receptor for an unknown ligand [55].

Expresion of PDGF β-receptor cDNA in CHO cells led to the synthesis of functionally active receptors [16, 44]. Subsequently, the structural and functional characteristics of mutated versions of the receptor have been analyzed with the aim of elucidating the structure-function relationship of the different domains of the receptor. An important question relates to the function of the kinase insert of the receptor. Receptor mutants in which the insert were deleted were able to transduce most of the early signals of PDGF such as phosphatidyl inositol turnover and c-*fos* expression, but did not mediate a mitogenic effect. Notably, the kinase activity of the mutated receptor was decreased and the substrate specificity altered, which suggest that it was unable to phosphorylate and activate a crucial substrate(s) in the mitogenic pathway [14, 45].

Substrates for the PDGF receptor kinases

Ligand binding induces autophosphorylation of both the PDGF α-receptor [21] and the β-receptor [13], as well as phosphorylation of cytoplasmic substrates [8, 12, 17]. It is likely that some of these substrates function in the signalling pathway and are activated after phosphorylation on tyrosine residues since β-receptors, in which the kinase activity has been extinguished by mutation of the ATP-binding lysine residue, is devoid of most of the activities associated with the receptor, such as stimulation of ion fluxes, gene expression, actin reorganisation, chemotaxis and mitogenicity [15, 53]. Some substrates of potential importance were recently identified, i. e. phosphatidylinositol 3' kinase [1], phospholipase C-γ [33, 50] and Raf-1, a serine/threonine kinase [34]. Phosphorylation of the two first substrates may mediate the stimulatory effect of PDGF on phosphatidyl-

inositol turnover. That Raf-1 may have an important function in the mitogenic pathway of growth factors, is indicated by the transforming properties
of aminoterminally trunctated constitutively activated Raf-1.

Activation by Dimerization of PDGF Receptors

Incubation of purified PDGF β-receptors with PDGF-BB lead to
dimerization of receptors as revealed by cross-linking experiments [3, 29].
Cross-linking occurred in a dose-dependent manner and decreased at
higher concentrations of PDGF-BB, suggesting that each subunit in the
dimeric ligand bind one receptor molecule [29]. Dimerization was found to
be closely associated with activation of the protein tyrosine kinase activity
of the receptor, measured as receptor autophosphorylation as well as phosphorylation of external substrates.

The structural similarity between the two PDGF receptor types suggests that the α-receptor also undergoes dimerization after binding of any
of its ligands (fig. 1). In order to explore the possibility that also heterodimeric receptor complexes can be formed, we took advantage of the observation that β-receptors, but not α-receptors, induce actin reorganization

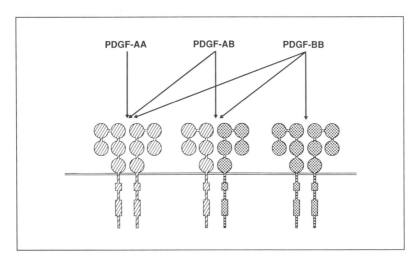

Fig. 1. Schematic illustration of the binding of the different isoforms of PDGF to
homo- and heterodimeric complexes of PDGF receptors. The receptors are drawn to indicate that they contain five extracellular immunoglobulin-like domains and an intracellular
split protein tyrosine kinase.

and membrane ruffling in human fibroblasts [35]. We found that in the presence of α-receptors, PDGF-AB induced actin reorganization, whereas in cells where the α-receptors had been blocked by an excess of PDGF-AA, or where the α-receptor was down-regulated by prior exposure to PDGF-AA at 37° C, the effect of PDGF-AB on actin reoganization was inhibited [20]. In fact, in the absence of α-receptors PDGF-AB acted as a β-receptor antagonist and inhibited the effect of PDGF-BB. We interpret these results to indicate that PDGF-AB activates the β-receptor by forming a heterodimeric receptor complex including one α- and one β-receptor molecule. Evidence for the existence of PDGF receptor heterodimers has also been obtained by co-precipitation studies [43].

Receptor dimerization has also been discussed in conjunction with activation of other receptors, such as the receptor for epidermal growth factor [42], and may be a general mechanism for growth factor-induced receptor activation.

Regulation of PDGF Receptor Expression in vivo

PDGF α- and β-receptors are expressed on many different normal and malignant cell types. Most normal cells with PDGF receptors have both types, but there are examples of cells having only α-receptors, i.e. o-2A glial progenitor cells of the rat opic nerve [24], or only β-receptors, i.e. capillary endothelial cells of the rat brain [47]. Analyses by Northern blotting have revealed that PDGF α- and β-receptor mRNA are expressed in an uncoordinated manner in many tumor cell lines of mesenchymal and glial origin [32; Nistér et al. unpublished; Leveen et al. unpublished].

The availability of monoclonal antibodies against PDGF β-receptors [38], has made possible immunohistochemical analysis of β-receptor expression in vivo. In contrast to the constitutive expression of β-receptors on connective tissue cells in vitro, β-receptors seem not to be expressed on most cells of normal tissues [49]. Receptors become expressed, however, on these cell types in conjunction with inflammation, such as in the synovium of patients with reumatoid arthritis [41]. Certain non-inflammatory tissues, such as the endometrium of the uterus, also contain cells with PDGF β-receptors [49]. Information about α-receptor expression in vivo is still not available.

The responsiveness to PDGF in vivo thus seems to be regulated at the level of receptor expression. In order to understand the role of PDGF in vivo, it will therefore be important to identify the factors that control PDGF receptor expression.

Future Perspectives

The recent information on PDGF and its receptors have unravelled a growth regulatory system of unexpected complexity. Three isoforms of PDGF, -AA, -AB and -BB, have been identified; in addition, the A chain occurs as two different variants due to differential splicing of the gene. The PDGF isoforms bind to at least two different receptor types and activate these by forming homo- or heterodimeric receptor complexes. There is evidence that at least one of the receptor types need to be induced on cells in vivo before these become responsive to PDGF stimulation.

Important directions of furture research include a better understanding of the similarities and differences of the functional activities of the two PDGF receptor types, the mechanism whereby they stimulate cell proliferation of cultured cells, and their in vivo function.

Acknowledgements

We thank Ingegärd Schiller for valuable help in the preparation of this manuscript.

References

1   Auger KR, Serunian LA, Soltoff SP, Libby P, Cantley LC: PDGF-dependent tyrosine phosphorylation stimulates production of novel polyphosphoinositides in intact cells. Cell 1989;57:167–175.
2   Betsholtz C, Johnsson A, Heldin CH, Westermark B, Lind P, Urdea MS, Eddy R, Shows TB, Philpott K, Mellor A, Knott TJ, Scott J: cDNA sequence and chromosomal localization of platelet-derived growth factor A-chain and its expression in tumour cell lines. Nature 1986;320:695–699.
3   Bishayee S, Majumdar S, Khire J, Das M: Ligand-induced dimerization of the platelet-derived growth factor receptor. Monomer-dimer interconversion occurs independent of receptor phosphorylation. J Biol Chem 1989;264:11699–11705.
4   Bonthron DT, Morton CC, Orkin SH, Collins T: Platelet-derived growth factor A chain: Gene structure, chromosomal location, and basis for alternative mRNA splicing. Proc Natl Acad Sci USA 1988;85:1492–1496.

5 Claesson-Welsh L, Eriksson A, Morén A, Severinsson L, Ek B, Östman A, Betsholtz C, Heldin CH: cDNA cloning and expression of a human platelet-derived growth factor (PDGF) receptor specific for B-chain-containing PDGF molecules. Mol Cell Biol 1988;8:3476–3486.

6 Claesson-Welsh L, Eriksson A, Westermark B, Heldin CH: cDNA cloning and expression of the human A type PDGF receptor establishes structural similarity to the B type PDGF receptor. Proc Natl Acad Sci USA 1989;86:4917–4921.

7 Claesson-Welsh L, Hammacher A, Westermark B, Heldin CH, Nistér M: Identification and structural analysis of the A type receptor for PDGF: Similarities with the B type receptor. J Biol Chem 1989;264:1742–1747.

8 Cooper JA, Bowen-Pope DF, Raines E, Ross R, Hunter T: Similar effects of platelet-derived growth factor and epidermal growth factor on the phosphorylation of tyrosine in cellular proteins. Cell 1982;31:261–271.

9 Coughlin SR, Escobedo JA, Williams LT: Role of phosphatidylinositol kinase in PDGF receptor signal transduction. Science 1989;243:1191–1994.

10 Coussens L, Van Beveren C, Smith D, Chen E, Mitchell RL, Isacke C, Verma IA, Ullrich A: Structural alteration of viral homologue of receptor protooncogene fms at carboxyterminus. Nature 1986;320:277–280.

11 Doolittle RF, Hunkapiller MW, Hood LE, Devare SG, Robbins KC, Aaronson SA, Antoniades HN: Simian sarcoma virus oncogene, v-sis, is derived from the gene (or genes) encoding a platelet-derived growth factor. Science 1983;221:275–277.

12 Ek B, Heldin CH: Use of an antiserum against phosphotyrosine for the identification of phosphorylated components in human fibroblasts stimulated by platelet-derived growth factor. J Biol Chem 1984;259:11145–11152.

13 Ek B, Westermark B, Wasteson Å, Heldin CH: Stimulation of tyrosine-specific phosphorylation by platelet-derived growth factor. Nature 1982;295:419–420.

14 Escobedo JA, Williams LT: A PDGF receptor domain essential for mitogenesis but not for many other responses to PDGF. Nature 1988;335:85–87.

15 Escobedo JA, Barr PJ, Williams LT: Role of tyrosine kinase and membrane-spanning domains in signal transduction by the platelet-derived growth factor receptor. Mol Cell Biol 1988;8:5126–5131.

16 Escobedo JA, Keating MT, Ives HE, Williams LT: Platelet-derived growth factor receptors expressed by cDNA transfection couple to a diverse group of cellular responses associated with cell proliferation. J Biol Chem 1988;263:1482–1487.

17 Frackelton AR Jr, Tremble PM, Williams LT: Evidence for the platelet-derived growth factor stimulated tyrosine phosphorylation of the platelet-derived growth factor receptor in vivo. Immunopurification using a monoclonal antibody to phosphotyrosine. J Biol Chem 1984;250:7909–7915.

18 Gronwald RGK, Grant FJ, Haldeman BA, Hart CE, O'Hara PJ, Hagen FS, Ross R, Bowen-Pope DF, Murray M: Cloning and expression of a cDNA coding for the human platelet-derived growth factor receptor: Evidence for more than one receptor class. Proc Natl Acad Sci USA 1988;85:3435–3439.

19 Hammacher A, Hellman U, Johnsson A, Gunnarsson K, Östman A, Westermark B, Wasteson Å, Heldin CH: A major part of PDGF purified from human platelets is a heterodimer of one A chain and one B chain. J Biol Chem 1988;263:16493–16498.

20   Hammacher A, Mellström K, Heldin CH, Westermark B: Isoform-specific induction
      of actin reorganization by platelet-derived growth factor suggests that the functio-
      nally active receptor is a dimer. EMBO J 1989;8:2489–2495.
21   Hammacher A, Nistér M, Westermark B, Heldin CH: The A-type receptor for plate-
      let-derived growth factor mediates protein tyrosine phosphorylation, receptor trans-
      modulation and a mitogenic response. Biochem J 1989;264:15–20.
22   Hart CE, Seifert RA, Ross R, Bowen-Pope DF: Synthesis, phosphorylation and
      degradation of multiple forms of the platelet-derived growth factor receptor studied
      using a monoclonal antibody. J Biol Chem 1987;262:10780–10785.
23   Hart CE, Forstrom JW, Kelly JD, Seifert RA, Smith RA, Ross R, Murray MJ, Bowen-
      Pope DF: Two classes of PDGF receptors recognize different isoforms of PDGF.
      Science 1988;240:1529–1531.
24   Hart IK, Richardson WD, Heldin CH, Westermark B, Raff MC: PDGF receptors on
      cells of the oligodendrocyte-type-2 astrocyte (o–2A) cell lineage. Development 1989;
      105:595–603.
25   Heldin CH, Westermark B: Growth factors as transforming proteins. Eur J Biochem
      1989;184:487–496.
26   Heldin CH, Westermark B: Platelet-derived growth factor: Three isoforms and two
      receptor types. Trends Genet 1989;5:108–111.
27   Heldin CH, Johnsson A, Wennergren S, Wernstedt C, Betsholtz C, Wasteson Å:
      A human osteosarcoma cell line secretes a growth factor structurally related to a
      homodimer of PDGF A chains. Nature 1986;319:511–515.
28   Heldin CH, Bäckström G, Östman A, Hammacher A, Rönnstrand L, Rubin K, Nistér
      M, Westermark B: Binding of different dimeric forms of PDGF to human fibroblasts:
      Evidence for two separate receptor types. EMBO J 1988;7:1387–1394.
29   Heldin CH, Ernlund AS, Rorsman C, Rönnstrand L: Dimerization of B type PDGF
      receptors occurs after ligand binding and is closely associated with receptor kinase
      activation. J Biol Chem 1989;264:8905–8912.
30   Hoppe J, Weich HA, Eichner W: Preparation of biologically active platelet-derived
      growth factor type BB from a fusion protein expressed in Escherichia Coli. Biochem
      1989;28:2956–2960.
31   Keating MT, Williams LT: Processing of the platelet-derived growth factor receptor.
      Biosynthetic and degradation studies using antireceptor antibodies. J Biol Chem
      1987;262:7932–7937.
32   Matsui T, Heidaran M, Miki T, Toru M, Popescu N, La Rochelle W, Kraus M, Pierce
      J, Aaronson SA: Isolation of a novel receptor cDNA establishes the existence of two
      PDGF receptor genes. Science 1989;243:800–803.
33   Meisenhelder J, Suh PG, Rhee SG, Hunter T: Phospholiphase C-γ is a substrate to
      the PDGF and EGF receptor protein tyrosine kinases in vivo and in vitro. Cell 1989;
      57:1109–1122.
34   Morrison DK, Kaplan DR, Escobedo JA, Rapp UR, Roberts TM, Williams LT: Direct
      activation of the serine/threonine kinase activity of Raf-1 through tyrosine phospho-
      rylation by the PDGF β-receptor. Cell 1989;58:649–657.
35   Nistér M, Hammacher A, Mellström K, Siegbahn A, Rönnstrand L, Westermark B, Hel-
      din CH: A glioma-derived PDGF A chain homodimer has different functional activities
      than a PDGF AB heterodimer purified from human platelets. Cell 1988;53:791–799.

36   Östman A, Rall L, Hammacher A, Wormstead MA, Coit D, Valenzuela P, Betsholtz C,
      Westermark B, Heldin CH: Synthesis and assembly of a functionally active recombinant
      PDGF-AB heterodiner. J Biol Chem 1988;263:16202–16208.
37   Östman A, Bäckström G, Fong N, Betsholtz C, Wernstedt C, Hellmann U, Westermark
      B, Valenzuela P, Heldin CH: Expression of three recombinant homodimeric isoforms of
      PDGF in Saccharomyces cerevisiae. Evidence for differences in receptor binding and
      functional activities. Growth Factors 1989;1:271–281.
38   Rönnstrand L, Terracio L, Claeson-Welsh L, Heldin CH, Rubin K: Characterization of
      two monoclonal antibodies against the external domain of the recpetor for platelet-deri-
      ved growth factor. J Biol Chem 1988;263:10429–10435.
39   Rorsman F, Bywater M, Knott TJ, Scott J, Betsholtz C: Structural characterization of the
      human platelet-derived growth factor A-chain cDNA and gene: Alternative exon usage
      predicts two different precursor proteins. Mol Cell Biol 1988;8:571–577.
40   Ross R, Raines EW, Bowen-Pope DF: The biology of platelet-derived growth factor. Cell
      1986;46:155–169.
41   Rubin K, Tingström A, Hansson GK, Larsson E, Rönnstrand L, Klareskog L, Claeson-
      Welsh L, Heldin CH, Fellström B, Terracio L: Induction of B-type receptors for platelet-
      derived growth factor in vascular inflammation: possible implications for development
      of vascular proliferative lesions. Lancet 1988; I:1353–1355.
42   Schlessinger J: The epidermal growth factor receptor as a multifunctional allosteric pro-
      tein. Biochem 1988;27:3119–3123.
43   Seifert RA, Hart CE, Philips PE, Forstrom JW, Ross R, Murray M, Bowen-Pope DF:
      Two different subunits associate to create isoform-specific platelet-derived growth factor
      receptors. J Biol Chem 1989;264:8771–8778.
44   Severinsson L, Claeson-Welsh L, Heldin CH: A PDGF B type receptor lacking most of
      the intracellular domain escapes degradation after ligand binding. Eur J Biochem 1989;
      182:679–686.
45   Severinsson L, Ek B, Mellström K, Claeson-Welsh L, Heldin CH: Deletion of the
      kinase insert of the B-type PDGF receptor affects receptor kinase activity and signal
      transduction. Mol Cell Biol 1990;10:801–809
46   Siegbahn A, Hammacher A, Westermark B, Heldin CH: Differential effects of the vari-
      ous isoforms of platelet-derived growth factor on chemotaxis of fibroblasts, monocytes
      and granulocytes. J Clin Invest 1990;85:916–920.
47   Smits A, Hermansson M, Nistér M, Karnushina I, Heldin CH, Westermark B, Funa K:
      Rat brain capillary endothelial cells express functional PDGF B-type receptors. Growth
      Factors 1989;2:1–8.
48   Stroobant P, Waterfield MD: Purification and properties of porcine platelet-derived
      growth factor. EMBO J 1984;3:2963–2967.
49   Terracio L, Rönnstrand L, Tingström A, Rubin K, Claeson-Welsh L, Funa K, Heldin
      CH: Induction of platelet-derived growth factor receptor expression in smooth
      muscle cells and fibrobasts upon tissue culturing. J Cell Biol 1988;107:1947–1958.
50   Wahl MI, Olashaw NE, Nishibe S, Rhee SG, Pledger WJ, Carpenter G: Platelet-deri-
      ved growth factor induces rapid and sustained tyrosine phosphorylation of phospho-
      lipase C-γ in quiescent BALB/c 3T3 cells. Mol Cell Biol 1989;9:2934–2943.
51   Waterfield MD, Scrace GT, Whittle N, Stroobant P, Johnsson A, Wasteson Å,
      Westermark B, Heldin CH, Huang JS, Deuel TF: Platelet-derived growth factor is

structurally related to the putative transforming protein p28^{sis} of simian sarcoma virus. Nature 1983;304:35–39.

52 Westermark B, Betsholtz C, Johnsson A, Heldin CH: Acute transformation by simian sarcoma virus is mediated by an externalized PDGF-like growth factor, in Kjelgaard NO, Forchhammer J (eds): Viral carcinogens. Copenhagen, Munksgaard 1987; pp 445–457.

53 Westermark B, Siegbahn A, Heldin CH, Claesson-Welsh L: The B type receptor for platelet-derived growth factor mediates a chemotactic response via ligand-induced activation of the receptor protein tyrosine kinase. Proc Natl Acad Sci USA 1990;87:126–130.

54 Yarden Y, Escobedo JA, Kuang WF Yang-Feng TL, Daniel TO, Tremble PM, Chen EY, Ando ME, Harkins RN, Francke U, Friend VA, Ullrich A, Williams LT: Structure of the receptor for platelet-derived growth factor helps define a family of closely related growth factor receptors. Nature 1986;323:226–232.

55 Yarden Y, Kuang WJ, Yang-Feng T, Coussens L, Munemitsu S, Dull TJ, Chen E, Schlessinger J, Francke U, Ullrich A: Human protooncogene c-kit: A new cell surface receptor tyrosine kinase for an unidentified ligand. EMBO J 1987;6:3341–3351.

C.-H. Heldin, Ludwig Institute for Cancer Research, Biomedical Center, P.O. Box 595, S-75123 Uppsala (Sweden)

Recessive Genetic Alterations

Contrib Oncol, vol 39, pp 125–134 (Karger, Basel, 1990)

p53 – Oncogene or Anti-Oncogene?

D. Eliyahu, D. Michalovitz, S. Eliyahu, O. Pinhasi-Kimhi, M. Oren

Department of Chemical Immunology, The Weizmann Institute of Science, Rehovot, Israel

p53 is a cellular phosphoprotein which has long been thought to be tightly associated with neoplastic transformation [5, 16, 17, 24, 27]. Furthermore, on the basis of studies by several laboratories it was proposed that p53 is an oncogene of the 'nuclear', *myc*-like type.

While there are many instances of p53 overproduction in transformed cells, there are other cases in which p53 expression is altogether absent. The best studied case is that of mouse spleen tumors induced by the Friend erythroleukemia virus [2, 4, 22, 23]. The detailed analyis of those tumors, many of which have no detectable normal p53 at all, has led to the suggestion that, in some cases, loss of normal p53 function may be advantageous for tumorigenesis. Recent studies involving human tumors lend further strong support to this idea [1, 19, 20, 30]. Hence, total absence or aberrant expression of p53 was found in a significant proportion of osteosarcomas, colorectal carcinomas, lung carcinomas and chronic myelogenous leukemias.

The apparent paradox of p53 having both a positive and a negative effect on transformation, became less surprising in light of the finding that wild-type (wt) p53 is devoid of any demonstrable transforming activity; the latter activity is exhibited only by plasmids carrying certain mutations in the protein [6, 11, 13, 14]. It was therefore conceivable that wt p53 may indeed interfere with transformation. In that case, the mutant p53 could promote transformation by blocking normal p53 function, acting in a dominant negative fashion [12].

To test this idea, we studied the effects of plasmids encoding wt p53 on the in vitro transformation of primary rat embryo fibroblasts (REF) [7]. REF can become neoplastically transformed through the combined action of plasmids overproducing mutant p53 and activated HA-*ras* [6, 9, 11, 13–15, 25]. If the transforming, mutant p53 plasmids were indeed working by interfering with the activity of wt p53, then one should be able to antagonize their transforming effects by increasing the amout of wt p53. We therefore studied the effect of various p53 plasmids on the transformation of REF by a combination of *ras* and pLTRcG9, which directs the abundant synthesis of mutant p53 [6]. To that end, a series of plasmids were constructed in which p53 expression was driven by the strong cytomegalovirus (CMV) immediate early enhancer-promoter [3]. The maps of these plasmids are shown in figure 1. pCMVNc9 expresses wt p53, whereas pCMVc5 encodes a

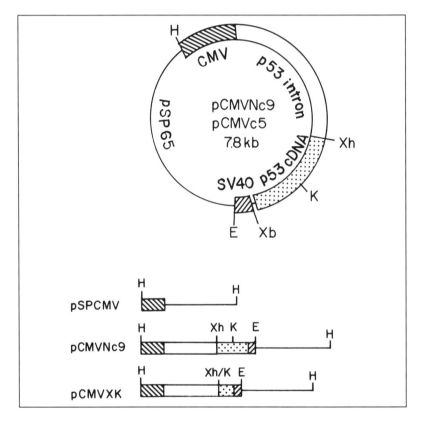

Fig. 1. p53 expression plasmids used in this study. Plasmids pCMVc5 and pCMVNc9 encode mutant and wild-type p53, respectively, under the control of the cytomegalovirus (CMV) immediate early enhancer-promoter element. pSPCMV contains only the CMV enhancer-promoter, while pCMVXK carries a deletion of the N terminal half of the p53 coding region (from the XhoI to the KpnI site); the remainder of the coding region is now placed out of phase with the correct reading frame (unpublished data). The origin of each DNA segment is indicated next to it. E-EcoRI; H-HindIII; K-KpnI; Xb-XbaI; Xh-XhoI.

mutant p53, carrying point mutations at the codons for amino acid 168 and 234 [6]. pSPCMV, containing vector sequences only, and pCMVXK (=pCMVp53d1), carrying a major deletion in the p53 coding region, served as negative controls. While pCMVc5 can also transform REF in concert with *ras*, its activity is much lower than that of pLTRcG9 (unpublished results).

The results of such an analysis are summarized in figure 2 (p53+*ras* columns). It is clear that inclusion of wt p53 plasmids in the assay led to a major reduction in the number of transformed foci induced by *ras* and pLTRcG9. In presence of pCMVNc9, there was a 25 fold decrease in the number of foci (from 10 per dish in the presence of the deleted plasmid to 0.4 per dish in the presence of pCMVNc9). No such effect was exerted by plasmid pCMVc5, encoding mutant p53. A transient expression experiment, employing REF, revealed that under these assay conditions pCMVp53wt made far less p53 than pLTRcG9. Yet, it was capable of very effectively inhibiting the transforming activity of the latter. This quantitative relationship strongly supports the notion that it is wt p53 that is functionally important in this system and argues against the possibility that the mutant is carrying a novel, dominant transforming activity.

The fact that the transforming activity of a mutant p53 gene can be efficiently abolished by plasmids encoding wt p53, supports the notion that

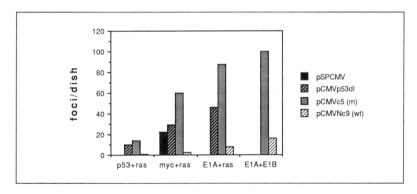

Fig. 2. Transformation of REF by different oncogenes in the presence of mouse p53 plasmids. Foci/dish values are averaged from several transfection dishes. The oncogene combinations employed for focus induction are indicated at the bottom. The p53 plasmids used for co-transfection with these oncogenes were as follows: pCMVc5, encoding a mutant p53 molecule with 2 amino acid substitutions; pCMVNc9, encoding wt p53; pCMVp53dl (referred to as pCMVXK in fig. 1) and pSPCMV (fig. 1) serving as a vector control.

mutant p53 plasmids act by interfering with the function of endogenous wt p53.

Non-established rat embryo fibroblasts can be very efficiently transformed by a combination of *ras* and plasmids encoding the *myc* protein [18]. To determine whether this process was also affected by the cellular levels of wt p53, we determined the effect of p53 plasmids on focus-induction by *myc*+ *ras*. As seen in figure 2, *myc+ras*-mediated transformation was also very sensitive to the presence of wt p53 expression plasmids. Inclusion of pCMVNc9 in the transformation mixture reduced the number of foci approximately 20 fold. Results of a tpyical experiment are presented in figure 3. Whereas several tens of foci are visible when pCMVXK (=p53dl) is added to the transfection mixture, there are almost no foci when pCMVNc9 (=p53wt) is included. When cell lines were established from foci generated in the presence of pCMVNc9, almost none expressed any detectable mouse p53. On the other hand, mouse p53 could easily be detected in almost all lines originating in *ras+myc*+pCMVc5 transfected cultures [7]. Hence, it seems likely that the few *myc+ras* transformants seen in the presence of

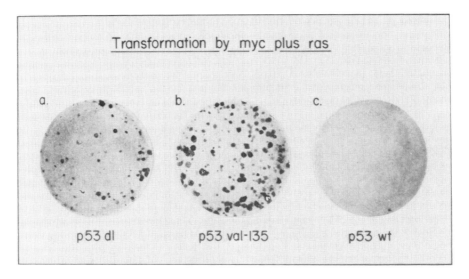

Fig. 3. Focus induction by *myc+ras* in the presence of different p53 plasmids. 90 mm dishes containing 8×10^5 cells were transfected with the indicated plasmid combinations, fixed and stained with Giemsa stain 9 days post-transfection. The different p53 plasmids included in the transfection mixtures are indicated at the bottom. p53 wt encodes wt 53, p53 Val-135 encodes a single amino acid substitution at residue 135, and p53 dl contains a large internal deletion in the p53 coding region.

pCMVNc9 represent cells in which this plasmid was either not present at all or inefficiently expressed. Interestingly, in most experiments there was a consistent enhancing effect on *myc+ras* transforming activity in the presence of plasmids encoding a mutant p53 (figure 2, pCMVc5 columns; figure 3, p53 Val-135). This could indicate a synergism between elevated *myc* expression and abrogated wt p53 activity in the transformation process.

The effect of wt p53 was next investigated in a system involving a viral oncogene, namely the adenovirus E1A gene. Like *myc*, E1A can also efficiently transform REF in concert with *ras* [28]. As can be seen in figure 2 (E1A+ras), pCMVNc9 exhibited a pronounced specific inhibitory effect also in this system. This particular plasmid combination also provided an additional advantage. The adenovirus plasmid used to express the E1A region, also contains part of the E1B region. Consequently, it can also transform REF in the absence of *ras* [28]. The resultant foci, however, develop much more slowly and are very different in morphology from the E1A+*ras* ones [28]. This provided the opportunity to study the effect of wt p53 on E1A+E1B-mediated transformation, in the absence of *ras*, by scoring pertinent typical foci at late times after transfection. As seen in Fig. 2 (E1A+ E1B) the wt p53 plasmid also greatly reduced the number of foci elicited by pLA8 alone. Thus, the inhibitory effect of excess wt p53 is not unique to *ras*-mediated focus induction.

In all the above experiments, wt p53 was found to inhibit the transformation of primary rat embryo fibroblasts. We next investigated the effect of the various p53 plasmids on established cells of the Rat-1 cell line. It was found [7] that while the growth of these cells was also adversely affected by wt p53 overproduction, the inhibition was much less dramatic than seen with oncogene-mediated transformation of REF. This fact argues against a general, non-selective 'toxic' effect of the wt p53 plasmids.

The results presented here, as well as similar recent findings by Levine and co-workers [10], raise the possibility that wt p53 may actually interfere with the progression of neoplastic processes, and thus qualify as an anti-oncogene. It should be kept in mind that all the observed inhibitory effects depend on the overproduction of wt p53 (CMV vectors), and hence may not precisely reflect the activities of wt p53 at physiological levels. Nevertheless, the fact that p53 is a frequent target for inactivation in human and rodent tumors lends strong support to the notion that p53 may indeed be an anti-oncogene also in vivo.

It is noteworthy that a mutant form of p53 which can interact with *ras* to transform REF [6], is at the same time devoid of the suppressor activity possessed by wt p53. This correlation has now been extended to two additional mutants, carrying point mutations at residues 135 and 215, respectively (unpublished data). Thus, there appears to be a linkage between loss of supressor activity and gain of apparent oncogenic activity in vitro. It is therefore significant that mutations in the same region of p53 are frequently found in human tumors [1, 30], and were interpreted to constitute loss of function mutants, missing a biochemical activity of wt p53 that is restrictive to neoplastic processes.

How can a loss-of-function mutant cooperate with *ras* in transformation and behave like a seemingly dominant oncogene? Clearly, such oncogenic activitiy by mutant p53 requires a great excess of the mutant p53 protein over the endogenous, presumably wt, p53, present in the REF. This is indicated by the fact that all lines generated from foci induced by *ras* + mutant p53 (at least those mutants tested so far) exhibit very high levels of the introduced p53 [6, 11, 13, 14]; our unpublished results). The large excess of biochemically inactive mutant p53 could interfere with the function of the endogenous counterpart simply by competition for common molecular targets. Another explanation is offered by the observation that in such mutant p53-transformed cells, practically all the endogenous p53 is tightly complexed with the transfected mutant protein [6]. Such a complex could either physically prevent the interaction of wt p53 with appropriate targets, or even result in its removal altogether into an inappropriate subcellular compartment.

These possibilities are illustrated in figure 4a. The inherent assumption is that the anti-oncogenic activity of p53, responsible for the inhibition of focus formation, involves the interaction of p53 with specific cellular targets (T). Mutations which abolish the ability of wt p53 to interact with such target will relieve its inhibitory effect (panel 2). When such mutant p53 is transfected into recipient cells (such as REF), it will also fail to interact with its specific target(s). Nevertheless, since the transfected cells continue to express also the endogenous wt p53, they may still provide an environment which is restrictive to transformation. If, however, the transfected mutant p53 can bind tightly the endogenous counterpart, and if it is present in a large enough excess, it can now interfere with the proper interaction of this endogenous wt p53 with its target(s). This, in turn, will abolish the transformation – inhibitory activity which is inherent to normal cells (panel 3).

So far, these models assume that the transforming variants of p53 are simple loss-of function mutants, and that there should be no difference between cells expressing such mutants and cells not expressing p53 at all.

While such interpretation is consistent with results obtained from the analysis of human [1, 30] and mouse [2, 4, 22, 23] tumors, there are other data suggesting that certain p53 mutants indeed possess a true dominant activity. The most striking case is that of the L12 mouse cell line, which is totally devoid of p53 expression [31]. Such cells are incapable of eliciting lethal tumors in syngeneic mice [26]. However, when transfected with a plasmid overexpressing mutant mouse p53, they now gain the capacity to cause aggressive, lethal tumors [32]. Hence, there must be a distinct activity that is contributed to L12 cells upon the introduction of mutant p53 overexpression.

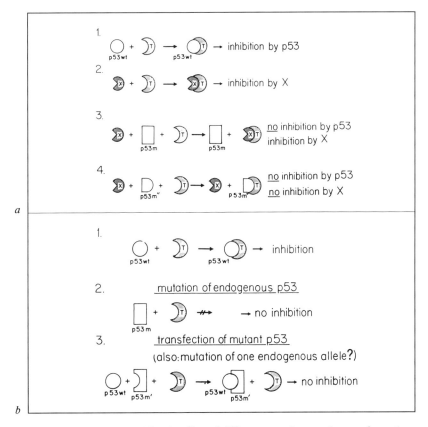

Fig. 4. a. b. Possible model for the effect of different mutations on the transformation-inhibitory activity of wt p53. T refers to a cellular p53 target with which p53 interacts, X refers to another cellular protein capable of interaction with target T. m, m′ and m″ denote different types of mutated p53 variants (see text).

A possible model which can account for these finding is depicted in figure 4b. The model assumes that the particular p53 target (T) responsible for its transformation-inhibitory effect (panel 1) can also interact with another protein (X), which would then be regarded as another hypothetical anti-oncogene. This interaction would also inhibit transformation (panel 2). Hence, if a cell contains a 'dead' p53 mutant (p53m), incapable of any molecular interaction, it may still be subject to inhibition by X (panel 3). The same may apply to cells in which no p53 is expressed at all. If, however, the p53 mutant (p53 m″) is capable of binding the target but can not activate it properly, it will still be able to block it and prevent protein X from interacting with it. In that case, no inhibition to transformation will be exerted by either p53 or protein X (panel 4). It is conceivable that L12 cells expressing a transfected mutant p53 represent such a case.

Finally, does the fact that wt p53 can inhibit neoplastic processes imply that it also plays a growth-inhibitory role in normal cells? Such a conclusion would seemingly conflict with earlier studies, which demonstrated that p53 expression is actually essential for ongoing cell proliferation, and that down-regulating p53 levels by either anti-p53 antibodies [21] or antisense transcripts [29] results in growth arrest. This conflict may be resolved by assuming that in normal cells, p53 acts within a tightly controlled chain of growth regulatory events. Blocking any of these steps in normal cells may abort the entire process and lead to inhibition of cell proliferation. On the other hand, when this pathway becomes grossly perturbed by events such as uncontrolled *myc* overexpression, p53 may in fact provide an inappropriate environment for transformation.

Despite the fact that the precise mode of action of p53 is practically unknown, our findings predict that loss of wt p53 function could provide a positive selective advantage in certain neoplastic processes. The recent evidence from various tumor systems is highly consistent with this notion.

Acknowledgements

We thank Dr. M. Horowitz and B. Fleckenstein for the generous gift of plasmids, and Ms. Esther Gross for secretarial assistance. This work was supported in part by grants from the Forchheimer Center for Molecular Genetics, the Minerva Foundation (Munich) and the Laub Foundation. M. Oren is a scholar of the Leukemia Society of America, Inc.

References

1   Baker SJ, Fearon ER, Nigro JM, et al: Chromosome 17 deletions and p53 gene mutations in colorectal carcinomas. Science 1989;244:217–221.

2   Ben-David Y, Prideaux VR, Chow V, et al: Inactivation of the p53 oncogene by internal deletion or retroviral integration in erythroleukemic cell lines induced by Friend leukemia virus. Oncogene 1988;3:179–185.

3   Boshart M, Weber F, Jahn G, et al: A very strong enhancer is located upstream of an immediate early gene of human cytomegalovirus. Cell 1985;41:521–530.

4   Chow V, Ben-David Y, Bernstein A, et al: Multistage Friend erythroleukemia: independent origin of tumor clones with normal or rearranged p53 cellular oncogene. J Virol 1987;62:2777–2781.

5   Crawford LV: The 53,000 cellular protein and its role in transformation. Int Rev Exp Pathol 1983;25:1–50.

6   Eliyahu D, Goldfinger N, Pinhasi-Kimhi O, et al: Meth A fibrosarcoma cells express two transforming mutant p53 species. Oncogene 1988;3:313–321.

7   Eliyahu D, Michalovitz D, Eliyahu S, et al: Wild-type p53 can inhibit oncogene-mediated focus formation. Proc Natl Acad Sci USA 1989;86:8763–8767.

8   Eliyahu D, Michalovitz D, Oren M: Overproduction of p53 antigen makes established cells highly tumorigenic. Nature 1985;316:158–160.

9   Eliyahu D, Raz A, Gruss P, et al: Participation of p53 cellular tumor antigen in transformation of normal embryonic cells. Nature 1984;312:646–649.

10   Finlay CA, Hinds PW, Levine AJ: The p53 proto-oncogene can act as a suppressor of transformation. Cell 1989;57:1083–1093.

11   Finlay CA, Hinds PW, Tan TH, et al: Activating mutations for transformation by p53 produce a gene product that forms an hsc70-p53 complex with an altered half-life. Mol Cell Biol 1988;8:531–539.

12   Herskowitz I: Functional inactivation of genes by dominant negative mutations. Nature 1987;329:219–222.

13   Hinds P, Finlay C, Levine AJ: Mutation is required to activate the p53 gen for cooperation with the *ras* oncogene and transformation. J Virol 1989;63:739–746.

14   Jenkins JR, Rudge K, Chumakov P, Currie GA: The cellular oncogene p53 can be activated by mutageneis. Nature 1985;317:816–818.

15   Jenkins JR, Rudge K, Currie GA: Cellular immortalization by a cDNA clone encoding the transformation-associated phosphoprotein p53. Nature 1984;313:651–654.

16   Jenkins JR, Stürzbecher HW: The p53 oncogene, in: Reddy EP, Skalka AM, Curran T (eds): The Oncogene Handbook. New York, Elsevier, 1988, pp 403–423.

17   Klein G: Advances in Viral Oncology, Vol. 2. The transformation-associated cellular p53 protein. New York, Raven Press, 1982.

18   Land H, Parada LF, Weinberg RA: Tumorigenic conversion of primary embryo fibroblasts requires at least two cooperating oncogenes. Nature 1983;304:596–602.

19   Lübbert M, Miller CW, Crawford LV, Koeffler HP: p53 in chronic myelogenous leukemia. J Exp Med 1988;167:873–886.

20   Masuda H, Miller C, Koeffler HP, et al: Rearrangement of the p53 gene in human osteogenic sarcomas. Proc Natl Acad Sci USA 1987; 84:7716–7719.

21   Mercer WE, Avignollo C, Baserga R: Role of the p53 protein in cell proliferation as studied by microinjection of monoclonal antibodies. Mol Cell Biol 1984;4:276–281.

22   Mowat MA, Cheng A, Kimura N, et al: Rearrangements of the cellular p53 gene in erythroleukemic cells transformed by Friend virus. Nature 1985;314:633–636.

23 Munroe DG, Rovinski B, Bernstein A, Benchimol S: Loss of a highly conserved domain on p53 as a result of gene deletion during Friend virus-induced erythroleukemia. Oncogene 1988;2:621–624.

24 Oren M: The p53 cellular tumor antigen; gene structure, expression and protein properties. Biochim Biophys Acta 1985;823:67–78.

25 Parada LF, Land H, Weinberg RA, et al: Cooperation between gene encoding p53 tumor antigen and *ras* in cellular transformation. Nature 1984;312:649–651.

26 Rotter V, Abutbul H, Wolf D: The presence of p53 transformation-related protein in Ab-MuLV transformed cells is required for their development into lethal tumors in mice. Int J Cancer 1983;31:315–320.

27 Rotter V, Wolf D: Biological and molecular analysis of p53 cellular encoded tumor antigen. Adv Cancer Res 1984;32:113–141.

28 Ruley HE: Adenovirus early region 1A enables viral and cellular transforming genes to transform primary cells in culture. Nature 1983;304:602–606.

29 Shohat O, Greenberg M, Reisman D, et al: Inhibition of cell growth mediated by plasmids encoding p53 anti-sense. Oncogene 1987;1:277–283.

30 Takahashi T, Nau MM, Chiba I, et al: p53: a frequent target for genetic abnormalities in lung cancer. Science 1989;246:491–494.

31 Wolf D, Admon S, Oren M, Rotter V: Abelson murine leukemia virus-transformed cells that lack p53 protein synthesis express aberrant p53 mRNA species. Mol Cell Biol 1984;4:552–558.

32 Wolf D, Harris N, Rotter V: Reconstitution of p53 expression in a nonproducer Ab-MuLV-transformed cell line by transfection of a functional p53 gene. Cell 1984; 38:119–126.

M. Oren, Department of Chemical Immunology,
The Weizmann Institute of Science, Rehovot 76100 (Israel)

Contrib Oncol, vol 39, pp 135–141 (Karger, Basel, 1990)

The Tumor Suppressor Gene *Lethal(3) Malignant Brain Tumor (1(3)mbt)* of *Drosophila Melanogaster:* Multiple Functions During Development

E. Gateff, T. Miyamoto

Institut für Genetik, Johannes-Gutenberg-Universität, Mainz, FRG

A number of tumor suppressor genes have been identified by genetic analysis in *Drosophila melanogaster* [3, 4]. The wild-type alleles of these genes are involved in the differentiation of specific cell-types. When homozygously mutated, malignant or benign tumors develop in defined cell-types or tissues. Six genes are known to cause benign ovarian – respectively ovarian and testis tumors. In five mutants lethality ensues at the end of larval life as a result of severe hematopoietic malignancies. Lethal imaginal discs tumors develop in three mutants. Finally three genes cause in the homozygous mutated state malignant transformation of the presumptive neuroblasts of the adult optic centers in the larval brain (for review on tumorsuppressor genes see [5]). Developmental aspects of one of the three mutants developing tumors in the adult optic centers of the larval brain, namely the *lethal(3)malignant brain tumor (1(3)mbt)* mutant, will be discussed in the following text.

Developmental Analysis of the 1(3)mbt^{ts-1} Mutant Animals

The cytogenetic locus of the *1(3)mbt* gene is on the right arm of the third chromosome in the region *97F* (T. Löffler and E. Gateff, unpublished results). We isolated three mutant *1(3)mbt* alleles. One of the three alleles, the *1(3)mbt*$^{ts-1}$ allele is temperature-sensitive.

At the permissive temperature of 22° C all homozygous mutant animals develop normally. However, when shifted to the restrictive temperature of 29° C with the onset of embryonic development, all late third instar larvae show a brain tumor and die around puparium formation. The tumors developing in the presumptive adult optic centers of the larval brain consists of adult optic neuroblasts and optic ganglion-mother cells, which, unable to differentiate, engage in an autonomous, invasive and lethal growth in situ as well after transplantation into a wild-type adult host [4]. The wild-type optic neuroblasts and ganglion-mother cells, in contrast, divide only a limited number of times before differentiating into adult optic neurons [8].

Thus, in the $1(3)mbt^{ts-1}$ mutant allele differentiation of the optic ganglion-mother cells into adult optic neurons obviously does not take place. Their unlimited capacity to divide cause a two to three fold increase of each brain hemisphere and their invasive behavior destroys the healthy portions of the larval brain.

Conditional mutants are useful tools to study the time of the gene expression and the phenotypes caused by the malfunctioning gene at the restrictive temperature. In a series of 'shift up' and 'shift down' experiments the time of development during which the $1(3)mbt$ gene has to be expressed in order differentiation of the adult optic neuroblasts and ganglion-mother cells to take place and tumor development to be suppressed was studied. The 'shift up' experiments performed in twelve hour intervals during embryonic and larval life showed an unusually long temperature-sensitive phase for tumor suppression. This period encompassed the entire embryonic stage, the first and almost the entire second larval instars. 'Shift up' experiments thereafter, e. g. during the late second and the third larval instars, did not impair the differentiation of the adult optic neuroblasts and ganglion-mother but resulted in female sterility (see later). Thus, in order for tumorous development to be suppressed and differentiation of the adult optic neuroblasts and ganglion-mother cells to take place the functional $1(3)mbt$ gene product has constantly to be present, during the above developmental period.

'Shift down' experiments during this time rescued the animals from developing a tumor. This findings allowed the conclusion that the temperature-sensitive $1(3)mbt^{ts-1}$ product regained its function quickly at the permissive temperature and, thus, prevented tumorous growth. When the time of development at the restrictive temperature extended into the third larval instar, 'shift down' experiments could no longer rescue the animals from developing a brain tumor. The results from the 'shift up' and 'shift down' experiments taken together indicate that at the end of the second and during the third larval instar the $1(3)mbt$ gene products is no longer needed for the differentiation of the adult optic neuroblasts and ganglion-mother cells. Thus, the established neoplastic growth proceeds autonomously at the restricitve as well as the permissive temperature. In addition to the malignant tumorous growth of the adult optic neuroblasts and ganglion-mother cells at the restrictive temperature, the development of the *l(3)mbt*[ts-1] imaginal discs is also impaired. Wild-type imaginal discs growth through larval life into blastemas of characteristic shapes and sizes [11]. The cells in the folded, monolayered imaginal disc epithelium are laterally connected with desmosomes and gap junctions and show an apical basal polarity which reflects their determination and future functions, namely to secrete the cuticular patterns of the adult integument.

The growth pattern of *l(3)mbt*[ts-1] imaginal discs at the permissive temperature of 22° C is identical to that of wild-type imaginal discs. At the restrictive temperature, however, the *l(3)mbt*[ts-1] imaginal discs appear smaller and exhibit malformations of their epithelial folding patterns. Histological preparations of mutant imaginal discs show monolayered arrangement of the cells. When tested for their developmental capacities by injection into ready to pupariate, wild-type larvae they differentiate into cuticular structures which, however, show bristle pattern abnormalities when compared with wild-type, metamorphosed imaginal disc implants. The temperature-sensitive period for developmental abnormalities of the imaginal disc coincides with that of the brain tumor.

The above observations show that the *l(3)mbt* gene product is also required for imaginal disc growth and differentiation. Its inactivation at the restrictive temperature causes, in contrast to the optic neuroblasts and ganglion-mother cells in the brain, no tumorous growth but defects in the adult integumental bristle and hair patterns.

'Shift up' experiments after the temperature-sensitive period for brain tumor development e. g. during the third larval instar and throughout adult development showed complete female sterility, indicating that the *l(3)mbt* function is also essential for oogenesis. The oogenesis defects, caused by the inactivation of the *l(3)mbt* gene at the restrictive temperature, are for the different developmental stages highly specific.

A short outline of wild-type oogenesis will precede the description and discussion of the defects in the mutant ovary observed in the different 'shift up' experiments. The fully grown wild-type ovary consist of approximately 16 elongated ovarioles. In the distal most portion of each ovariole, in the germarium, 2 – 3 oogonia are present. They divide to produce new oogonia and so called cystoblasts [9]. Each cystoblast produces by incomplete cytokinesis two cystocytes which remain interconnected via a ring canal. The three following, synchronous cell divisions yield a syncitial cyst of 16 cysto-cytes. A first stage egg chamber forms when, at the base of the germarium, the cyst becomes enveloped by a monolayer of follicle cells. With the entry of the egg chambers into the vitellarium a complex differentiation process, encompassing 13 developmental stages, ensues leading to the mature egg [9].

In the 'shift up' experiments $1(3)mbt^{ts-1}$ animals and wild-type controls were shifted to the restrictive temperature in 12 h intervals during the 24 h long 3rd larval instar and throughout adult development in the pupa which lasts about five days. The ovaries of the eclosed mutant adults were investigated anatomically as well as histologically and their defects were compared to that of the wild-type controls. In the 'shift up' experiments during the third larval instar oogenesis was arrested predominantly at the cystocyte stage. Egg chambers were not present in the ovaries of the flies at eclosion. Shifts arount the time of puparium-formation and 12 h thereafter, showed in the ovaries of the adults at eclosion few first stage egg chamber. In contrast to the wild-type, however, these egg chambers did not develop into mature eggs but degenerated. In shifts between 24 and 60 h after pupariation oogenesis proceeded to the vitellogenesis stage. The formed eggs were shorter and degenerated before they could be layed. The shifts at 72 and 84 h after pupariation showed in the ovaries eggs of normal appearance which, however, did not develop beyond the blastoderm stage. In the shifts 24 h before eclosion of the flies from the puparium a maternal effect was observed. The embryos reached the segmentation stage. All embryos showed, however head defects. In addition to the head defects approximately 40 % of the embryos exhibited dorsal integumental defects. 'Shift down' experiments restored the fertility of the mutant female flies. In the wild-type controls at the restrictive temperature oogenesis and embryogenesis proceeded normally.

Discussion

The 'shift up' and 'shift down' experiments presented here demonstrated that the $1(3)mbt$ gene plays a vital role in the differentiation of at least three cell-types and tissues, namely the presumptive adult optic neuroblasts and ganglion-mother cells in the larval brain, the imaginal discs and the female germ-line. In these three tissues the $1(3)mbt$ mutation causes different developmental defects. In the female germ-line the absence of a functional *l(3)mbt* gene product interferes with virtually all main differentiation stage, such as, cystocyte division, cyst- and egg chamber formation, vitellogenesis and the realization of maternal messages. The lack of *l(3)mbt* function in the imaginal discs, on the other hand, does not interfere with the capacity of the cells to secrete a cuticle. The secreted cuticle, however, exhibits highly abnormal hair- and birstle- patterns. In the adult optic neuroblasts and ganglion-mother cells the lack of *l(3)mbt* gene function prevents entirely their differentiation and, thus, is responsible for their malignant neoplastic growth.

Until the cloning of the gene and its molecular analysis only speculations can be forwarded concerning the differential mode of action, of the *l(3)mbt* gene product in the three cell- and tissue-types. Since the *l(3)mbt* gene function is required throughout development the assumption can be made that the gene product engages in multiple interactions, either directly with genes as a regulatory protein or with a network of stage- and cell-specific regulatory factors which together determine individual differentation steps. In the absence of the ubiquitous *l(3)mbt* gene product the interactions with these stage- and cell-specific factors do not take place and, thus, abnormally differentiation is arrested or proceeds.

In *Drosophila* most mutated genes, including the tumor-suppressor genes, cause more or less severe pleiotropic effect [5]. For instance, the animals carrying the *lethal(2)giant larvae (1(2)gl)* mutation show, in addition to brain- and imaginal disc-tumors, also abnormalities in the fat bodies, the salivary- and ring glands [5], which indicates multiple functions of the *l(2)gl* gene during development in the different cell- and tissue-types.

Among the many *Drosophila* genes with multiple functions during development two will briefly be discussed here. The *hairy (h)* gene product is instrumental in regulating both, embryonic segmentation as well as the establishment of the adult bristle pattern [6, 7, 10]. The two *h*-functions are developmentally regulated by the same *h*-protein which most probably is a transcription factor [12]. The interaction(s) of the *h* gene product with as yet unknown stage- and cell-specific factors may be responsible for its differential function during embryonic segmentation and as well as later during adult development when the secretion of the cuticular bristle pattern by the imaginal discs is underway.

Another example of a *Drosophila* gene with multiple functions during development is *daughterless (da)* [2]. *da* is expressed during oogenesis as a maternal message. Mutant *da/da* flies crossed with wild-type males lack daughters in their progeny. *da* is further an essential zygotic gene for both sexes. *da* deficient embryos lack their entire peripheral nervous system and parts of their central nervous system. Genetic data demonstrated further the interaction between *da* and genes of the *achaete scute complex (AS-C)*, which likewise affect the differentiation of the peripheral nervous system and are also involved in sex determination. Independent biochemical studies showed *da* and the genes of the *AS-C* to belong to a family of proteins which bind DNA via a *helix-loop-helix* motiv (*HLH*). Moreover, the function of *da* in sex-determination and dosage compensation was recently established [2]. The many functions of the *da* gene are presently regarded as stage- and tissue-specific interactions of the *HLH*-containing *da*-protein with the *HLH*-containing gene products of the *AS-C* and other genes [1, 2].

The ubiquitous *1(3)mbt* gene product is also envisioned to interact with stage- and cell-specific regulatory factors during the development. The inactivation of the *1(3)mbt*$^{ts-1}$ gene product at the restrictive temperature and, thus, the stage- and cell-specific interactions should reveal the function of this gene in tumor suppression as well as its role in promoting the differentiation of the imaginal discs, the female germ-line and the segmentation of the embryo.

References

1   Cline TW: Evidence that *sisterless-a* and *sisterless-b* are two of several discrete 'numerator elements' of the *X/A* sex determination signal in Drosophila that switch *Sxl* between two alternative stabel expression states. Genetics 1988;119:829 – 862.

2   Cline TW: The affairs of *daughterless* and the promiscuity of developmental regulators. Cell 1989;59:231 – 234.

3   Gateff E: Malignant neoplasms of genetic origin in the fruit fly *Drosophila melanogaster*. Science 1978;200:1446 – 1459.

4   Gateff E: Cancer, Genes and Development – the Drosophila Case? in Weinhouse S, Klein G. (eds): Advances in Cancer Research. London, Academic Press, 1982, vol 37, pp 33 – 69.

5   Gateff E, Mechler BM: Tumor-suppressor genes of *Drosophila melanogaster*. Crit Rev Oncogenesis 1989;1:221 – 241.

6   Ingham PW, Howard KR, Ish-Horowicz D: Transcription pattern of the *Drosophila* segmentation gene *hairy*. Nature 1985;318:439 – 445.

7   Ingham PW, Pinchin SM, Howard KR, Ish-Horovicz D: Genetic analysis of the *hairy* locus in *Drosophila*. Genetics 1985;111:463 – 486.

8   Kanckel DR, Ferrus A, Garren SH, Harte PJ, Lewis PE: The structure and development of the nervous system, in Ashburner M, Wright TRF (eds): The genetics and biology of drosophila. New York, Academic Press, 1980, vol 2d, pp 295 - 368.

9   King RC: Ovarian development in *Drosophila melanogaster*. New York, Academic Press, 1970, pp 1–17.

10 Nüsslein-Vollhard C, Wieschaus E: Mutations altering segment number and polarity in *Drosophila melanogaster*. Nature 1980;287:795–801.

11 Poodry CA: Imaginal discs: Morphology and development, in Ashburner M, Wright TRF (eds): The genetics and biology of drosophila. New York, Academic Press, 1980, vol 2d, pp 407–441.

12 Rushlow CA, Hogan A, Pinchin SM, Howe KM, Lardelli M, Ish-Horovicz D: The *Drosophila hairy* protein acts in both segmentation and bristle patterning and shows homology to *N-myc*. EMBO J 1989;8:3095–3103.

E. Gateff, Institut für Genetik, Johannes Gutenberg Universität,
Saarstraße 21, D-6500 Mainz (FRG)

Contrib Oncol, vol 39, pp 142–150 (Karger, Basel, 1990)

Wilms' Tumour – A Developmental Anomaly

V. van Heyningen, K. Pritchard-Jones, D. J. Porteous, W. Bickmore,
N. Hastie

MRC Human Genetics Unit, Western General Hospital, Edinburgh, UK

It is becoming an increasingly accepted concept that in the development of cancer cumulative stepwise DNA level changes in somatic cells lead to progressive loss of growth control and finally malignancy. The mutations survive precisely because they lead to proliferative advantage in progeny cells. Childhood tumours where the age-specific incidence peaks in early life may be expected to require fewer mutational steps than late onset malignancies. Another hallmark of several childhood cancers is that they virtually never present later in life, suggesting that the target cell population disappears with age, as the developmental program to adult form is completed.

With an incidence of 1 in 10,000, Wilms' tumour or nephroblastoma is the most common childhood solid tumour. Along with the paradigmatic early-onset neoplasm retinoblastoma, it is widely regarded as an embryonal cell malignancy [1]. Like retinoblastoma, a proportion of nephroblastomas are bilateral and a few (1 %) are familial. Statistical comparison of the retinoblastoma incidence curves for sporadic unilateral versus familial and bilateral tumours led to the two-step mutational hypothesis which was soon extended to the less clear-cut data for Wilms' tumour [2]. Most Wilms' tumours are sporadic, unilateral and without reported associated anomalies. However, as often happens, it is the rare cases with accompanying malformations that give insight into the genetics and biology of tumour development. The systematic histological survey of Wilms' tumour [3] has also contributed much to current understanding of the relationship between normal kidney development and the genesis of nephroblastoma.

How Genetics Can Lead to an Appreciation of Gene Function

The Two-step Hypothesis and Tumour Suppressor Genes – Lessons from the Paradigm

The two step hypothesis [2] for the development of retinoblastoma and nephroblastoma suggested that two mutational events are sufficient for the onset of malignancy. The earlier presentation of bilateral and familial cases in comparison with sporadic unilateral ones occurs because in the former categories there is a pre-existing germline of very early embryonic mutation and only one further hit is required before tumour development is seen. In the latter cases both mutations have to take place within the same somatic cell. This hypothesis could also explain the occurrence of non-penetrance, seen only rarely in familial retinoblastoma, but more frequently in cases where there is a known predisposition to Wilm's tumour.

The occasional observation of the same chromosomal deletion on cytogenetic analysis of retinoblastoma tumour material and in rare familial cases where there was accompanying mental retardation, placed the site of the retinoblastoma gene *(RB)* at chromosome 13q14 [4]. The fact that chromsomal *deletion* was involved, and the subsequent finding on molecular analysis of homozygous deletion of this region in occasional retinoblastomas, suggested that the changes involved in tumour development were homozygous loss-of-function mutations. This in turn meant that two hits must knock out both allelic sites at the single tumor predispositon locus. The loss of constitutional heterozygosity, frequently seen in tumours for markers known to be linked to the tumour locus, is good indication that the second functional allele is being lost in tumorigenesis [5]. With the cloning of the *RB* gene (see refs. in [6]) these predictions were eventually borne out [7].

Suppressor Gene Function

Connection war also made between the idea of a recessive tumour gene and the concept of tumour suppressor functions whose existence had been predicted from analysis of malignancy by cell fusion [8]. Both the *RB* gene and the Wilms' tumour predisposition gene *(WT)* are expected to exhibit suppressor activity in appropriate malignant cells – an expectation partly borne out for *RB* [9]. As far as *WT* is concerned, suppression of tumorigenicity in somatic cell hybrids has been observed in several malignant × normal cell combinations with retention of part or all of chromosome 11 (see below) [10]. It remains to be demonstrated that any *WT* candidate gene alone can fulfill this suppressor function.

Progress Towards the Isolation of the Wilms' Tumour Gene

The chromosomal location of the Wilms' tumour predisposition gene *(WT)* was first suggested by the observation that Wilms' tumour was accompanied by aniridia (absence of iris) at much higher than expected frequencies (see refs in [11]). On cytogenetic examination a high proportion of such individuals, often with other associated anomalies including mental retardation and genitourinary abnormalities – hence WAGR syndrome, were found to be hemizygous for a deletion which always included band p13 on chromosome 11. It became clear that a considerable number of patients with large deletions failed to present with Wilms' tumour, showing that there is only about 60 % penetrance for the progress to malignancy. Penetrance was also clearly reduced in the rare familial nephroblastoma cases (no deletions seen in any of these). With the aid of deletion mapping in a large collection of patients with complete or partial WAGR syndrome the position of the *WT* gene was increasingly finely defined by the combined efforts of several groups. Complete genetic and hence biological independence of aniridia from Wilms' tumour was demonstrated by mapping studies [12]. Intensive efforts toward isolating candidate *WT* genes included the whole armoury of techniques now being developed for reverse genetics: exhaustive cloning of small chromosomal regions, long range mapping, cloning from preparative pulsed field gels, chromosome walking and jumping as well as more biological approaches such as searching for homozygously deleted tumour material using new clones closer and closer to the putative *WT* locus [13 – 16]. The same gene, with characteristics compatible with those expected for *WT*, has now been isolated, reputedly in at least three different laboratories.

Biological Conclusions From Tumour Histology and From Associated Anomalies

Normal Kidney Development

Normal metanephric kidney development is initiated early in fetal life (35 days in man, 11 days in mouse), after mesonephric structures had already superseded the earliest non-functional pronephros. Mesenchymal metanephric blastemal elements condense around the bifurcating epithelial ureteric bud and differentiate into nephrons consisting of glomeruli and tubules, designed to collect excretory waste, reabsorb water and unused nutrients, and conduct it via the ureters to the bladder. This process of metanephric proliferation and differentiation produces the lobar structure of the mature kidney with the earliest produced nephrons nearest the medulla and the latest ones near the cortex.

Tumour-associated Histological Abnormalities

Normally blastemal elements should have disappeared by the time of birth in man, yet persistence of renal blastema in normal portions of the tumour-bearing kidney, or in the contra-lateral organ, is frequently seen in patients with Wilms' tumour. This persistence of nephrogenic rests (NR) has been carefully analyzed by Beckwith et al. [3] in the large series of tumour samples submitted for the US National Wilms' Tumor Survey (NWTS). The earliest onset tumours are most frequently associated with intralobar nephrogenic rests (ILNR) situated in the earliest developing regions [3, 17]. Later onset tumours display a higher frequency of perilobar nephrogenic rests (PLNR) in the newest cortical areas.

Developmental Anomalies Associated with Wilms' Tumour

As mentioned earlier, WAGR patients, particularly boys, frequently exhibit genital anomalies, predominantly bilateral cryptorchidism and hypospadias [11, 15, 17]. Occasionally the more extreme XY gonadal dysgenesis is seen [18]. However, these anomalies are not confined to WAGR and are also observed in association with sporadic Wilms' tumour with no visible cytogenetic abnormality. More rarely genital tract malformations are seen in female [46, XX] patients.

Abnormalities in kidney and urinary tract development are also frequently observed in individuals with Wilms' tumour. These anomalies include absent, fused or duplicated kidneys, abnormal ureters, as well as multicystic dysplastic kidneys [17]. In Drash syndrome [19], early onset kidney failure, often with mesangial sclerosis, is frequently associated with Wilms' tumour presenting in very young, karyotypically XY individuals with gonadal dysgenesis. Both Drash syndrome and WAGR-associated tumours are early onset and present a histological picture with ILNR [3].

Wilms' tumour is also by far the most frequent malignancy associated with Beckwith-Wiedemann syndrome (BWS), which is a developmental anomaly involving fetal overgrowth, sometimes presenting asymmetrically as hemihypertrophy [20]. Occasionally hemihypertrophy is the sole developmental abnormality seen in nephroblastoma cases. This category of overgrowth-associated tumours tend to be late onset and histologically showing PLNR.

The Relationship Between Developmental Anomalies and Genetics

The Lessons From Gene Mapping and Studying Normal Development

Most of the Wilms' tumour-associated developmental anomalies described above have also been observed in rare single instances in individuals with aniridia, with no nephroblastoma, suggesting that loss of gene(s) in the p13 region of chromosome 11 are implicated in their genesis. However, examination of the WAGR deletion map reveals that cryptorchidism/hypospadias map within the small (c. 350 kb) DNA segment which forms the smallest region of overlap for *WT* and which also happens to coincide with the region that is absent in a rare homozygous deletion case. Might it be possible that these abnormalities of male genital tract development are caused (with incomplete penetrance) by the same mutations which predispose to the development of Wilms' tumour? Such a pleiotropic effect for the *WT* gene would not be totally surprising, if we consider the developmental origin of the Wolffian duct which gives rise to vas deferens. It arises from the remnants of the mesonephric duct, which also gives rise to the ureteric bud around which metanephric blastemal condensation leads to the development of the mature kidney. Histological analysis of Wilms' tumour suggests that abnormal proliferation and differentiation of the blastemal elements occurs in kidneys before, or in parallel with, the development of malignancy. Aberrant control of proliferation and differentiation is the hallmark of malignancy. A gene normally involved in controlling the switch from stem cell proliferation to differentiation is an ideal candidate for an embryonal-cell tumour-predisposition locus.

Does the Candidate Gene Fit the Expected Characteristics?

Rumour has it that three separate laboratories have isolated what appears to be the same candidate for the *WT* gene. It maps to the SRO region defined by deletion mapping and within an even smaller homozygous deletion recently identified. We have been pleased to have collaborative access to the first version, cloned in the laboratory of David Housman [21]. The expression pattern by RNA blot hybridization shows the gene to be transcribed in fetal kidney, testis, ovary, spleen, and to a lesser extent in adult kidney. RNA in situ hybridization is beginning to reveal regional expression within the developing kidney. Sequence analysis revealed the presence of some 'zinc finger' homology in this gene [21], in good agreement with its putative function encoding a control element.

RNA bloot analysis of mRNA from a large number of tumours has revealed only normal sized message although large variation in relative expression levels has been seen. The search for point mutations is yet to be carried out.

Is This a Complete Answer to the Search for the WT Gene?

Loss of constitutional heterozygosity for chromosome 11p polymorphic markers in a large collection of tumours revealed that in a third of informative cases allele loss was confined to 11p15 markers. In such cases there is no evidence for two-step mutation at the 11p13 *WT* locus. Unexpectedly these cases include two instances of WAGR deletion individuals with allele loss at 11p15 only [22]. Familial BWS has been mapped to the p15 region of chromsome 11 [23, 24]. BWS has also been associated with partial trisomy for the 11p15 region. Is there at this site a second Wilms' tumour predisposition locus working by a different mechanism, but capable of interacting with the loss of function at 11p13 to produce a tumour?

Linkage analysis of rare pedigrees with familial Wilms' tumour showed that these nephroblastoma cases do not segregate with chromosome 11p13 or p15 markers [25, 26]. Do these results herald the existence of a third *WT* locus?

Can we, in addition, cope with the complication that when DNA from the parents of Wilms' tumour patients is available then in all but one instance out of more than 30 informative cases examined, the allele lost in the course of tumorigenesis is the maternal allele [e. g.: 27], suggesting that the first hit arises in the paternal genome which may be differentially imprinted [28, 29] for expression of the *WT* gene.

Another unexplained finding has been that among the offspring of nearly 100 survivors of unilateral Wilms' tumour, which should include at least some individuals with a germ line first hit, no offspring with nephroblastoma have been observed [30].

Clearly, even with a candidate gene cloned, there is a long way to go before we can claim a full understanding of the biology and genetics of Wilms' tumour and its relationship to normal kidney development.

References

1   Mierau GW, Beckwith JB, Weeks DA: Ultrastructure and histogenesis of the renal tumors of childhood: an overview. Ultrastruct Pathol 1987;11:313–333.
2   Knudson AG, Strong LC: Mutation and cancer: a model for Wilms' tumor of the kidney. J Natl Cancer Inst 1972;48:313–324.
3   Beckwith JB, Kiviat NB, Bonadio JF: Nephrogenic rests, nephroblastomatosis, and the pathogenesis of Wilms' tumor. Ped Pathol 1990;10:1–36.
4   Dryja TP, Rapaport JM, Joyce JM, Petersen RA: Molecular detection of deletions involving band q14 of chromosome 13 in retinoblastomas. Proc Natl Acad Sci USA 1986;83:7391–7394.
5   Cavenee WK, Dryja TP, Phillips RA, Benedict WF, Godbout R, Gallie BL, Murphree AL, Strong LC, White RL: Expression of recessive alleles by chromosomal mechanisms in retinoblastoma. Nature 1983;305:779–784.
6   Hansen MF, Cavenee WK: Retinoblastoma and the progression of tumor genetics. Trends Genet 1988;4:125–128.
7   Dryja TP, Mukai S, Petersen R, Rapaport JM, Walton D, Yandell DW: Parental origin of mutations of the retinoblastoma gene. Nature 1989;339:556–558.
8   Harris H: The analysis of malignancy by cell fusion: the position in 1988: Cancer Res 1988;48:3302–3306.
9   Huang HJS, Yee JK, Shew JY, Chen PL, Bookstein R, Friedmann T, Lee EYHP, Lee WH: Suppression of the neoplastic phenotype by the replacement of the RB gene in human cancer cells. Science 1988;242:1563–1566.
10 Weissman BE, Saxon PJ, Pasquale SR, Jones GR, Geiser AG, Stanbridge EJ: Introduction of a normal chromosome 11 into a Wilms' tumor cell line controls its tumorigenic expression. Science 1987;236:175–180.
11 van Heyningen V, Boyd PA, Seawright A, Fletcher JM, Fantes JA, Buckton KE, Spowart G, Porteous DJ, Hill RE, Newton MS, Hastie ND: Molecular analysis of chromosome 11 deletions in aniridia-Wilms tumor syndrome. Proc Natl Acad Sci USA 1985;82:8592–8596.
12 Davis LM, Stallard R, Thomas GH, Couillin P, Junien C, Nowak NJ, Shows TB: Two anonymous DNA segments distinguish the Wilms' tumor and aniridia loci. Science 1988;241:840–842.

13 Compton DA, Weil MM, Jones C, Riccardi VM, Strong LC, Saunders GF: Long range physical map of the Wilms' tumor-aniridia region on human chromosome 11. Cell 1988;55:827–836.

14 Lewis WH, Yeger H, Bonetta L, Chan HSL, Kang J, Junien C, Cowell J, Jones C, Dafoe LA: Homozygous deletion of a DNA marker from chromosome 11p13 in sporadic Wilms tumor. Genomics 1988;3:25–31.

15 Bickmore WA, Porteous DJ, Christie S, Seawright A, Fletcher JM, Maule JC, Couillin P, Junien C, Hastie ND, van Heyningen V: CpG islands surround a DNA segment located between translocation breakpoints associatd with genitourinary dysplasia and aniridia. Genomics 1989;5:685–693.

16 Gessler M, Thomas GH, Couillin P, Junien C, McGillivray BC, Hayden M, Jaschek G, Bruns GAP: A deletion map of the WAGR region on chromosome 11. Am J Hum Genet 1989;44:486–495.

17 Breslow N, Beckwith JB, Ciol M, Sharples K: Age distribution of Wilms' tumor: report from the National Wilms' Tumor Study. Cancer Res 1988;48:1653–1657.

18 Rajfer J: Associaton between Wilms' tumor and gonadal dysgenesis. J Urol 1981; 125:388–390.

19 Manivel JC, Sibley RK, Dehner LP: Complete and incomplete Drash syndrome: a clinicopathologic study of five cases of a dysontogenetic-neoplastic complex. Hum Pathol 1987;18:80–89.

20 Wiedemann HR: Tumours and hemihypertrophy associated with Wiedemann-Beckwith syndrome. Eur J Pediatr 1983;141:129.

21 Call KM, Glaser TM, Ito CY, Buckler AJ, Pelletier J, Haber DA, Rose EA, Kral A, Yager H, Lewis WH, Jones CA, Housman DE: Descripiton and characterization of a zinc fincer polypeptide gene at the human chromosome 11 Wilms' tumor locus. Cell 1989; in press.

22 Henry I, Grandjouan S, Couillin P, Barichard F, Huerre-Jeanpierre C, Glaser T, Philip T, Lenoir G, Chaussain JL, Junien C: Tumor-specific loss of 11p15.5 alleles in del 11p13 Wilms' tumor and in familial adrenocortical carcinoma. Proc Natl Acad Sci USA 1989;86:3247–3251.

23 Ping AJ, Reeve AE, Law DJ, Young MR, Boehnke M, Feinberg AP: Genetic linkage of Beckwith-Wiedemann syndrome to 11p15. Am J Hum Genet 1989;44:720–723.

24 Koufos A, Grundy P, Morgan K, Aleck KA, Hadro T, Lampkin BC, Kalbakji A, Cavenee WK: Familial Wiedemann-Beckwith syndrome and a second Wilms' tumor locus both map to 11p15.5. Am J Hum Genet 1989;44:711–719.

25 Huff V, Compton DA, Chao LY, Strong LC, Geiser CF, Saunders GF: Lack of linkage of familial Wilms' tumour to chromosomal band 11p13. Nature 1988;336:377–378.

26 Grundy P, Koufos A, Morgan K, Li FP, Meadows At, Cavenee WK: Familial predisposition to Wilms' tumour does not map to the short arm of chromosome 11. Nature 1988;336:374–376.

27 Schroeder WT, Chao LY, Dao DD, Strong LC, Pathak S, Riccardi V, Lewis WH, Saunders GF: Nonrandom loss of maternal chromosome 11 alleles in Wilms' tumors. Am J Hum Genet 1987;40:413–420.

28 Reik W, Surani MA: Genomic imprinting and embryonal tumours. Nature 1989; 338:112.

29 Sapienza C: Genome imprinting an dominance modification. Ann NY Acad Sci
     1989;564:24:38.
30 Li FP, Williams WR, Gimbere K, Flamant F, Green DM, Meadows AT: Heritable
     fraction of unilateral Wilms tumor. Pediatrics 1988;81:147–149.

V. van Heyningen, MRC Human Genetics Unit, Western General Hospital,
GB-Edinburgh, EH4 2XU (UK)

Contrib Oncol, vol 39, pp 151–156 (Karger, Basel, 1990)

Genetic Events in Development of Multiple Endocrine Neoplasia Type 2

B. Ponder

CRC Human Cancer Genetics Research Group, Department of Pathology, University of Cambridge, Great Britain

Multiple endocrine neoplasia type 2 (MEN 2) is an inherited cancer syndrome which consists of malignant tumours of the 'C' cells of the thyroid (medullary carcinoma of the thyroid, MTC) and usually benign tumours of the adrenal medulla (phaeochromocytoma) [1]. 10–40 % of individuals also have parathyroid hyperplasia or adenomas, which is of interest because although the 'C' cells and adrenal medulla are of neuro-ectodermal origin, the parathyroids are not.

MEN 2 has 3 clinical varieties, which breed true in families. They differ in age at onset, aggressiveness of the tumours, and in the presence of additional phenotypic abnormalities. In the commonest variety, MEN 2A, clinical onset is generally aged 40–50 (though there is wide variation) [2] and about 1/3 of those who present with clinical symptoms die of tumour. In MEN 2B, onset is younger and the tumours are more aggressive. There is also a characteristic phenotype which includes disorganised proliferation of peripheral somatic and autonomic nerve tissue, especially in the lining of hollow viscera: these tissues are also of neuroectodermal derivation. Parathyroid involvement in MEN 2B is said to be minimal or absent. The third variety, 'MTC-only', consists of a small number of large families in which there is no evidence of phaeochromocytoma, and in which the thyroid tumours present late and have an indolent course [3].

The inherited mutation for MEN 2A has been mapped by genetic linkage to the pericentromeric region of chromosome 10 [4]. Preliminary data suggest that MEN 2B and MTC-only may map to the same region [5, 6]. Several genetic events have been identified in the progression of MTC and phaeochromocytoma from patients with MEN 2A and MEN 2B, and in the non-hereditary forms of the same tumours. These include losses of heterozygosity on chromosomes 1p, 13q and 22. So far as the limited data allow, they seem to be similar for phaeochromocytoma and MTC, and for hereditary and non-hereditary forms [7 - 10].

The MEN 2 syndromes thus pose several questions of biological interest: (1) what is the nature of the germlinemutation? (2) Are the MEN 2A, MEN 2B and MTC-only mutations allelic at the same locus, and if so, how do the mutations determine the different disease phenotypes? (3) Why, if they share the same initial and subsequent mutations, are MTC malignant and phaeochromocytoma usually benign? (4) What are the putative suppressor genes involved in the losses of heterozygosity on chromosomes 1p and 22, and do the similar losses in other tumours of neuroectodermal origin (neuroblastoma, meningioma, schwannoma, melanoma) [11 - 13] involve the same genes, which might in that case be genes with a normal function specific to the neuroectodermal lineage?

The germline mutation for MEN 2

Because the families are large and more numerous, most of the data relate to MEN 2A. The MEN 2A locus has been mapped in a 3 centimorgan interval between the loci defined by pTB14.34 and IRBP, which lie either side of the centromere on chromosome 10 [4]. Studies of the entire family set by several groups have so far failed to reveal any recombinants between MEN 2A and the centromere itself, defined by the probe pα10RP8. The MEN 2A locus therefore lies close to the centromere, but whether on the short arm or the long arm is not known.

The germline mutation could involve either (1) loss of activity of the MEN 2A gene, or (2) an alteration of activity with the acquisition of new properties. By analogy with other inherited cancer syndromes such as retinoblastoma and familial polyposis coli, a loss of activity mutation might be expected: and again there are two possibilities. In retinoblastoma, loss of both alleles at the Rb locus is necessary for tumourigenesis. In familial polyposis loss of the second allele appears to be a late event, and the germline hemizygous loss is sufficient to cause the phenotype of abnormal epithelial proliferation and polyp formation, which suggests a dosage effect [14].

These three possibilities should in principle be distinguishable for MEN 2 as they have been in the other inherited cancer syndromes, by analysis of DNA from tumour, and of constitutional DNA and chromosomes from affected individuals, for evidence of deletions. In 42 MEN 2-related tumours informative with markers on the short and long arm of chromosome 10, we have found only 1 case of loss of heterozygosity [7, 8], involving the loss of the whole chromosome. Other groups report similar findings (2/16 [9] and 1/9 [10] losses). Cytogenetic studies of blood lymphocytes from unrelated MEN 2A and 2 MEN 2B patients in our own laboratory and reported by other groups [15, 16] have shown no abnormality in the pericentromeric region of chromosome 10.

The interpretation remains open. (1) MEN 2 may be a loss of function mutation with a requirement for somatic loss of the remaining wild-type allele, as in retinoblastoma. The second event in tumours may not have been detected because the proximity of the MEN 2 locus to the centromere leads to a low frequency mitotic recombination (which is an easily detectable mechanism of loss of heterozygosity), or possibly because hemizygous loss of another gene close to MEN 2 places cells at a selective disadvantage. (The frequent occurrence of chromosome 10 losses in gliomas [17] argues against this, but possibly these losses are tolerated in a different cell type or at a later stage of tumour progression than we are considering for MEN 2). (2) MEN 2 may be a loss of function mutation, where hemizygous loss alone has a phenotypic effect. In this case, the C-cell hyperplasia which is the characteristic precursor to MTC in hereditary cases would be the direct manifestation of the germline mutation, similar to the situation in familial polyposis of the colon. In this case, however, non-hereditary tumours might be expected to show loss of heterozygosity representing the initial event: but we found none. (3) The MEN 2 mutation may be an 'altered function' mutation. In this case, MEN 2 would differ from the inherited cancer syndromes for which the genetic mechanism is known [14]; but the apparently consistent finding of loss of function mutations in the syndromes elucidated thus far may simply be because the associated deletions and loss of heterozygosity are easy to detect, rather than necessarily implying that all will turn out to share the same mechanism.

MEN 2 is unusual among the inherited cancer syndromes in having at least 2 clearly distinct genetic forms (MEN 2A and MEN 2B) that map to the same genetic locus. Other syndromes also show considerable variation in expression (e. g. the Gardner's syndrome variant of familial polyposis) but in these cases variation seems to occur within as well as between families, and so it cannot so confidently be ascribed to differences in the germline mutation. Two questions arise about the relationship of the germline MEN 2 mutation to the disease phenotype. (1) Assuming the MEN 2A and MEN 2B mutations are allelic, then if the mutation involves loss of gene activity, it is clear that it cannot be a complete loss in each case, or there should be no phenotypic differences between them. Analogy with Duchenne and Becker muscular dystrophy suggests that the MEN 2B mutation will usually be the more extensive in its effects, although this does not necessarily imply a more extensive genomic deletion [18]. The parathyroid involvement in MEN 2A and lack of it in MEN 2B is hard to explain on this model: an alternative is to postulate that the different MEN 2 syndromes involve deletion of different combinations of several adjacent genes [19]. (2) There is a consensus in the literature, supported by our own data (unpublished), that the thyroid tumours in MEN 2B are not only of earlier onset, but also more aggressive in behaviour. The earlier onset can easily be ascribed to a stronger stimulus in MEN 2B to C-cell hyperplasia, and so the earlier development of the target cell population from which the tumours will arise. The patterns of metastatic behaviour and growth of an established tumour, however, are more usually ascribed to genetic events in tumour progression. It is less obvious how these are influenced by the nature of the initial mutation.

Events in tumour progression

We have concentrated on a search for consistent patterns of loss of heterozygosity in tumours, which may indicate the chromosomal locations of suppressor genes, losses of which are involved in tumour progression. Our results to date, almost entirely based on primary tumour material, are summarised in table 1. The losses on chromosomes 1p, 13q and 22 are

Table 1. Loss of heterozygosity in sporadic and familial MEN 2-related tumours

	MTC		Phaeochromocytoma	
	sporadic	MEN 2	sporadic	MEN 2
Chromosome				
1p	0/3	7/16	2/6	1/3
10	0/6	1/22	0/9	0/5
22	0/1	1/10	1/2	1/1
Other chromosomes	0/38	1/133	1/45	1/17

The figures are number of losses / number of informative comparisons.
The chromosomes involved in losses other than 1p, 10 and 22 were : 3p, 5q and 7p

above the very low background 'noise' of losses on other chromosomes, and are therefore presumably significant events in tumour progression. With one exception (a non-hereditary phaeochromocytoma which showed LOH on chromosome 22) every tumour that showed LOH on a chromosome other than chromosome 1, also showed LOH on chromosome 1p. This suggests that the 1p losses may occur at a relatively early stage. There are, however, few data yet on the stage at which these events occur, on their relationship to the histological differentiation or prognosis of the tumour, or to other events such as n-myc amplification, which has been reported in C-cell hyperplasia [20], or oncogene activation. Systematic comparisons between metastases and primary tumour also have still to be done. Other tumours of neuroectodermal origin show fequent losses of heterozygosity or cytogenetic changes affecting chromosomes 1p and 22. Abnormalities of these chromosomes also occur quite commonly in cancers of non-neuro-ectodermal origin, so the observations must be interpreted with caution until the loci involved in each case have been precisely defined. It is, however, an interesting possibility that the occurrence of genetic events on chromosomes 1p and 22 in different neuroectodermal tumours may point to a small number of loci on these chromosomes which have a normal role in the growth and differentiation of neuroectodermal lineages.

Acknowledgements

I thank my numerous collaborators in this work, whose contribution is recognised by their authorship of the primary papers referred to in the text. The work in Dr. Ponder's laboratory is supported by the Cancer Research Campaign.

References

1   Thakker RV, Ponder BAJ: Multiple endocrine neoplasia, Clinical Endocrinology and Metabolism. London, Balliere Tindall, 1989; Vol 2, No 4, pp 1031–1067.
2   Easton DF, Ponder MA, Cummings T, et al: The clinical and screening age-at-onset distribution for the MEN 2 syndrome. Am J Hum Genet 1989;44:208–215.
3   Farndon JF, Dilly WG, Baylin SB, et al: Familial medullary thyroid carcinoma without associated endocrinopathies: A distinct clinical entity. Br J Surg 1986; 73:278–281.
4   Nakamura Y, Mathew CGP, Sobol H, et al: Linked markers flanking the gene for multiple endocrine neoplasia type 2A. Genomics 1989;5:199–203.

5   Jackson CE, Norum RA, O'Neal LW, et al: Linkage between MEN 2B and chromosome 10 markers linked to MEN 2A. Am J Hum Genet 1988;43:A147.

6   Noll WW, Bowden DW, Maurer LH, et al: Genetic mapping of familial medullary carcinoma of the thyroid/multiple endocrine neoplasia 2A with polymorphic loci on chromosome 10. Am J Hum Genet 1988;43:A29.

7   Landsvater RM, Mathew CGP, Smith BA, et al: Development of multiple endocrine neoplasia type 2A does not involve substantial deletions of chromosome 10. Genomics 1989;4:246–250.

8   Ponder BAJ, Smith BA, Marcus EM, et al: Genetic events in tumourigenesis in multiple endocrine neoplasia type 2. Cancer Cells 1989;7:219–221.

9   Nelkin BD, Nakamura Y, White RW, et al: Low incidence of loss of chromosome 10 in sporadic and hereditary human medullary thyroid carcinoma. Cancer Res 1989; 49:4114–4119.

10 Takai S, Tateishi H, Nishisho I, et al: Loss of genes on chromosome 22 in medullary thyroid carcinoma and phaeochromocytoma. Jpn J Cancer Res 1987;78:894–898.

11 Fong C-T, Dracopoli NC, White PS, et al: Loss of heterozygosity for the short arm of chromosome 1 in human neuroblastoma: correlation with n-myc amplification. Proc Natl Acad Sci USA 1989;86:3753–3757.

12 Seizinger BR, Rouleau G, Ozelius LJ, et al: Common pathogenetic mechanism for three tumour types in bilateral acoustic neurofibromatosis. Science 1987;236:317–319.

13 Dracopoli NC, Harnett P, Bale SJ, et al: Loss of alleles from the distal short arm of chromosome 1 occurs late in tumour progression. Proc Natl Acad Sci USA 1989; 86:4614–4618.

14 Ponder BAJ: Gene losses in human tumours. Nature 1988;335:400–401.

15 Wurster-Hill DH, Noll WW, Bircher LY, et al: A cytogenetic study of familial medullary carcinoma of the thyroid. Cancer Res 1986;46:2134–2138.

16 Fletjer WL, Babu VC, Van Dyke DL, Jackson CE: High resolution studies of chromosome 10 in 23 MEN-2 families. Cancer Genet Cytogenet 1988; 32:301–303.

17 Fujimoto M, Fults DW, Thomas GA, et al: Loss of heterozygosity on chromosome 10 in human glioblastoma multiforme. Genomics 1989;4:210–213.

18 Monaco AP, Bertelson CJ, Liechti-Gallati S, et al: An explanation for the phenotypic differences between patients bearing partial deletions of the DMD locus. Genomics 1988;2:90–95.

19 Talpos GB, Jackson CE, Toyy JB, Van Dyke DL: Phenotypic mapping of the multiple endocrine neoplasia type II syndrome. Surgery 1983;94:650–654.

20 Boultwood J, Wyllie FS, Williams ED, Wynford-Thomas D: N-myc expression in neoplasia of human thyroid C-cells. Cancer Res 1988;48:4073–4077.

B. Ponder, CRC Human Cancer Genetics Research Group, Dept. of Pathology, University of Cambridge, Tennis Court Road, Cambride CB2 1QP (UK)

Diagnostic Aspects

Contrib Oncol, vol 39, pp 157–168 (Karger, Basel, 1990)

Genetic Basis for Tumor Progression

W. K. Cavenee

Ludwig Insitute for Cancer Research, Royal Victoria Hospital,
Montreal, Quebec, Canada

Two important realizations about the group of diseases collectively termed cancer have become prominent over the past two decades. The first point is that traditional therapeutic approaches work well, but often only in very specific instances. The phenomenology upon which this statement is based is of two types. For example, some highly defined tumors, such as testicular cancers or hairy cell leukemias, respond extraordinarily and almost uniformly well to therapies whereas some tumors, like glioblastoma multiforme, are virtually unresponsive. Other tumor classes, like carcinoma of the breast, include cases that respond well and others that do not. A joint consideration of these clinical observations could suggest that therapies are best designed for tumors that are best defined and that classes with mixed respones are, in fact, composed of two subclasses which have dramatically different prognoses.

The second realization is that cancer is largely a disease elicited by genetic alterations. In human populations, three types of clinical observation provide circumstantial, but often paradoxical, support for this idea. Firstly, specific types of tumors can occur in families with behavior consistent with the the transmission of a Mendelian autosomal dominant predisposition. This presentation is reasonably easy to understand for single and homogeneous tumors but much less so when several types of seemingly unrelated tumors appear to be the phenotypic manifestation of the trait. Secondly, individuals with a well-defined initial cancer occurrence can often develop a second primary tumor of a different histological type in a distinct body site. Finally, individuals with a variety of multiorgan developmental defects can be at greatly increased risk for the development of specific, often rare, tumor types. If these tumors are rare, a statistical argument can be forwarded that such an occurence is so unlikely that it suggests an etiological relationship.

These observations are even more perplexing in light of the large body of evidence indicating that the neoplastic process requires the accumulation of several events and that many of these may comprise specific chromosomal rearrangements. One way to view the problem is that the somatic nature of most cancer requires that these genetic abnormalities be acquired during the replication of cells from the specifically affected organ. Perhaps the most likely cellular function to blame for their occurrence is the process of mitotic duplication and segregation of chromosomes from progenitor to daughter cells. Of course, many aberrations in this process would be expected to be lethal while others would confer no particular selective advantage. The rare events comprising viable, advantageous and transforming mitotic abnormalities could conceivably represent the molecular underpinnings of the neoplastic process. Further, the inheritance of aberrations which are uncovered by mitotic errors might have organismal effects responsible for some of the paradoxical population characteristics of cancer. This hypothesis is particularly attractive in the case of the association of developmental organismal anomalies with the high risk for rare tumors.

In this paper, I will review the efforts my colleagues and I have made in the past few years to apply molecular genetics to the question of the specificity of these genetic lesions to the process of cancer predisposition and progression. It is our hope that uncovering the nature and function of such defects will lead to the more appropriate allocation of therapies as well as, perhaps, the development of new targetted approaches.

Loss of Genetic Information in Cancer Predisposition and Progression

In experimental chemical carcinogenesis, the earliest event in tumorigenesis is termed the initiating event. In the human population such initiations may be transmitted as inherited predisposition. At least fifty different forms of human cancer have been observed to aggregate in families as well as to have corresponding sporadic forms. Obviously, these individuals represent a valuable resource in attempts to define the targets of initial genotoxic damage. In many of these cases the aggregation occurs with a pattern consistent with the transmission of an autosomal dominant Mendelian trait. This interpretation is, however, at odds with three lines of evidence. First, if a single mutation was sufficient in and of itself to elicit a tumor, then families segregating for autosomal dominant forms of cancer would be expected to have no normal tissue in the diseased organ. This expectation is in direct contrast to the clinical observation of discrete tumor foci amidst normal, functional tissue in such individuals. Secondly, elegant epidemiological analyses [1] of sporadic and familial forms of several cancer types have indicated that the conversion of a normal cell to a tumor cell requires multiple events. Finally, there is a substantial body of evidence derived from somatic cell hybrids which indicates dominance of the wild type phenotype in the presence of tumorigenic mutations [2].

In brief, one can consider the development of cancer to be the clonal evolution of cells which have undergone a series of genetic alterations which confer growth advantages at specific stages in the process outlined in figure 1a [3]. Our work over the past few years has been directed at defining these genetic events. In particular, we have taken advantage of the prescient observations of Knudson [1] which suggested the requirement for as few as two mutations to elicit the entry of a precursor cell into the neoplastic pathway. In this model, hereditary cases have inherited a germinal mutation which does not, in itself, cause the tumor but rather predisposes each precursor cell to a further transforming event. In this model, the nonhereditary cases would also result from two mutations except that these events would have to occur in the same somatic cell. Thus, the two forms of the disease could be viewed as resulting from the same two-step process, at the level of the aberrant cell, the difference being the inheritance or somatic occurence of the first mutation.

We proposed [4] that the second step in tumorigenesis in both heritable and sporadic tumors involves somatic alteration of the normal allele at the "tumor locus' in a way that unmasks the mutant allele. Thus, the first mutation in this process, although it may be inherited as an autosomal dominant trait at the organismal level would be expected to have the properties of a recessive defect at the level of the individual retinal cell. In this model, (fig. 1b) the heritable form of the disease arises as a germinal mutation of the *TMR* locus and is inherited by an individual who, therefore, is an obligate heterozygote (t/+) at the *TMR* locus in each of his somatic and germ cells. A subsequent event in any of his target cells which results in homozygosity for the mutant allele (that is, mutant at the *TMR* locus on both chromosome homologues) will result in a tumor clone. The chromosomal mechanisms which could accomplish this loss of constitutional heterozygosity include: mitotic nondisjunction with loss of the wild-type chromosome, which would result in hemizygosity at all loci on the chromosome, mitotic nondisjunction with duplication of the mutant chromosome which results in homozygosity at all loci on the chromosome; or mitotic

A.

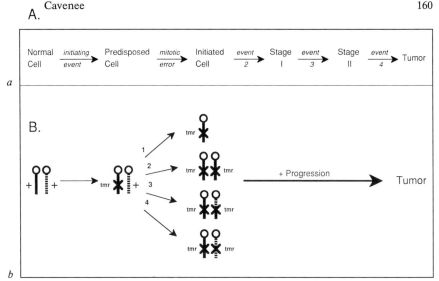

a

b

Fig. 1. a. Accumulation of genetic damage culminates in malignancy. The pathway can initiate in a single somatic cell in sporadic cases or in any cell in heritable cases. *b.* A model for chromosomal mechanisms which can accomplish the conversion of a normal cell to a cell that is homozygous for inactivation of a tumor (TMR) locus. Predisposition occurs either by inheritance or by somatic occurence of a mutation which converts a wild-type (+) allele to an inactive allele (TMR). A tumor could then occur by elimination of the remaining wild-type allele by nondisjunction (1), nondisjunction/duplication (2), mitotic recombination (3) or regional aberration (4). Additional genetic damage is required for the progression of homozygously defective cells to frank neoplasia.

recombination between the chromosomal homolgues with a breakpoint between the *TMR* locus and the centromere, which would result in hetero-zygosity at loci in the proximal region and homozygosity throughout the rest of the chromosome including the *TMR* locus. Regional events such as gene conversion, deletion, or mutation must also be considered. Heritable and sporadic retinoblastoma could each arise through the appearance of homozygosity at the *TMR* locus, the difference being two somatic events in the sporadic case as compared to one germinal and one somatic event in the heritable case.

The test of this hypothesis was first made with the childhood eye tumor, retinoblastoma. We compared alleles at loci on various chromo-somes in tumor and normal tissues from affected individuals; such loci are defined by restriction fragment length polymorphism. We have examined a large series of cases of retinoblastoma in this way and these relatively gross chromosomal mechanisms appear to be involved in about 75 %. Further-more, the notion that these chromosomal gymnastics serve to uncover pre-disposing cellular recessive mutations was strongly supported by the demonstration that, in familial cases, the chromosome remaining in the tumor was inherited from the affected parent [5].

This approach to uncovering genetic alterations which have occurred early enough to comprise monoclonal characteristics of the tumor has been extended to a variety of human tumor types with a remarkable degree of success (table 1). Virtually every type examined has shown regions of the tumor genome which have become homozygous. These include common and rare cancers, diseases which affect primarily children or adults, and neoplasias of almost every ontogeny from which human cancer can arise. The data in most of these cases can be fit to the model outlined in figure 1 such that predispositions that are somatically recessive first undergo homo-

Table 1. Losses of heterozygosity in human tumors

Chromosome Region	Tumors
1p	neuroplastoma, melanoma, breast carcinoma, pheochromocytoma, medullary thyroid carcinoma
2	uveal melanoma
3p	renal cell carcinoma, testicular, small cell lung carcinoma, uterine carcinoma
5q	colon carcinoma
10	glioblastoma
11p	Wilm's tumor, embryonal rhabdomyosarcoma, hepatoblastoma, adrenal carcinoma, breast carcinoma, transitional cell bladder carcinoma, hepato-cellular carcinoma, testicular tumors.
11q	insulinomas, parathyroid tumors
13q	retinoblastoma, osteosarcoma, small cell lung carcinoma, breast carcinoma, hepatocellular carcinoma.
14q	neuroblastoma
17p	colon carcinoma, breast carcinoma, osteosarcoma, small cell lung carcinoma, astrocytoma
18q	colon carcinoma
22	acoustic neuroma, meningioma

zygosis and then are compounded by genotoxic damage which leads to increasingly malignant phenotypes. The concerted losses of alleles at loci on several chromosomes in some tumors (e.g. breast carcinoma, colon carcinoma and small cell lung carcinoma) likely suggest that losses of heterozygosity play a role in later stages of malignant progression as well.

Clinically Associated Cancers

The model shown in figure 1 predicts that genomic aberration will be cumulative throughout the process of malignancy. Such aberrations can be recessive or dominant mutations, amplification of genes for growth factors or their receptors, as well as acquired cellular aggression characteristics. Such events comprising homozygosity of chromosome 17p, amplification of the epidermal growth factor receptor and chromosome 10 hemizygosity do appear to occur (or be selected for) in a specific order in brain tumors [6, 7] but the model does not require this to be so. In fact, a similar accumulation of genetic aberrations has been uncovered in the transition of normal colonic epithelium to adenomatous polyps to colon carcinoma [8]. Thus, although these data are only correlative at present, the identification of these nonrandom events may serve as the beginning of a genotypic, rather than phenotypic, approach to the definition of the molecular underpinnings of human tumor predisposition and progression.

The foregoing discussion has been limited to consideration of a unilinear variation of the original model of Nowell [3] and the mechanistic involvement of genotoxic damage and chromosomal rearrangement in the process. There is, of course, no reason that more than one progressional event could not occur in different cellular derivatives of an irreversibly committed precursor. Such a consideration is schematically outlined in figure 2. This variation of the model predicts that cells of different lineages might give rise to their cognate tumors through common predisposition. Since any initiating mutation would likely be occurring with a low probability the chance of similar or identical mutations taking place in two unrelated tissues of the same person would seem vanishingly small. Thus, the search for support for the idea might most effectively begin by identification of inherited mutations which effect syndromes that encompass more than one tumor type. From an experimental point of view, confidence in the approach would be considerably enchanced if the syndrome and the tumors were rare individual occurrences in the general population so as to trivialize the possibility of chance associations.

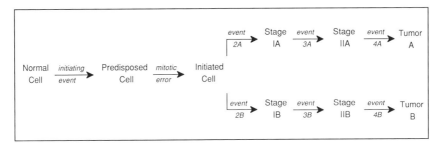

Fig. 2. Tumors of different types could arise subsequent to a common predisposing mutation if progressional damage of different types is either tissue-specific in effect or elicits differentiation along two different lineages.

Here, I will discuss one example of a syndrome characterized by developmental malformations and high risk for the development of specific rare tumors. The Beckwith-Wiedemann syndrome (BWS) is a congenital disorder consisting of developmental anomalies with associated neoplastic disease. The developmental anomalies are characterized by excess growth at the cellular adrenal cortical cytomegaly), tissue (pancreatic, renal, and pituitary hyperplasia), organ (macroglossia, hepatomegaly), whole body segment (hemihypertrophy), or even whole body (gigantism) levels. Other characteristics of the syndrome include omphalocele or umbilical hernia, facial flame nevus, renal medullary dysplasia, and hypoglycemia that may be secondary to pancreatic islet cell hyperplasia. Of particular interest for this discussion is the fact that more than 10 % of all individuals with BWS will develop rare cancers, including Wilms' tumor, hepatoblastoma, rhabdomyosarcoma and adrenal carcinoma [9] in association with the growth excess disorders which characterize the syndrome. Although most cases of BWS are sporadic, several instances of apparent autosomal dominant inheritance have been described [10] albeit with reduced penetrance and variable expressivity. Cytogenetic examination of constitutional cells from children with BWS has sometimes shown structural abnormalities of chromosome 11 including duplication of the 11p13-p15 region [11] and duplication of 11p15 only. The significance of these observations lies in their implication of the short arm of chromosome 11 as a likely location for at least one of the genes involved in the syndrome. In fact, genetic linkage analysis supports this conclusion: familial predisposition to the syndrome segregates with loci in the 11p15.5 region of the genome [12]. It is a reasonable assumption, then, that tumors might arise in BWS patients by fixation of predisposition in somatic cells by attainment of functional homozygous defectiveness for a locus in 11p15.5, as proposed in figure 3. Further, it could be envisaged that additional progressional events which differed in homozygous kidney, liver, striated muscle, or adrenal cortex could give rise to distinct tumor types in the same individual, a proposal concordant with clinical evidence ([9], Y. Tsunematsu and S. Watanabe, personal communication). The experimental expectation is that, whatever the accumulated progressional differences between the tumors, the initial predisposition should be held in common. Further, sporadic forms of the tumors should share these initial events, at least in a proportion of cases. In order to test this hypothesis, we examined allelic combination at loci on chromosome 11p in the tumors associated with the syndrome: Wilms' tumor [13] rhabdomyosarcoma [14, 15], and hepatoblastoma [14].

Wilms' tumor, a neoplasm of embryonal kidney, exhibits several features analogous to those previously discussed for retionoblastoma: constitutional deletions of chromosome region 11p13 appear to predispose to the disease [16]; chromosome 11 abnormalities involving the same region are frequent in tumor tissue; and sporadic and inherited autosomal dominant forms have been described [17]. These cases imply that mutant forms of one or more loci contained within the 11p13 band predispose to tumor development but are not sufficient to elicit the cancer because discrete tumor foci are seen amidst a background of normal kidney, even in cases in which the 11p13 band of one homologue is missing in the germline. Thus, a second, postzygotic, event appears to be required as well.

In order to determine whether chromosomal mechanisms similar to those described above for retinoblastoma play a role in the development of Wilms' tumor, DNA samples from normal and tumor tissues were analyzed for their genotypic combinations at loci on chromosome 11 [13]. Examples of the data are shown in table 2a and indicate loss of germline alleles, which seemed to arise by chromosomal loss and duplication, in the majority of tumors. Similar results were obtained in three other laboratories, as well [18–20]. A likely explanation for these results, based on previous work with retinoblastoma, is that mitotic segregation ovents occurred in each predisposed kidney cell such that one chromosome homologue was lost and the remaining homologue was duplicated during the process of tumorigenesis. We infer that the remaining chromosomes are each defective at the Wilms' tumor locus on chromosome 11p. Evidence in support of this idea was provided by the introduction of a normal chromosome 11 into Wilms' tumor cells by microcell transfer [21]. The resulting hybrid cells lost the ability to

Table 2. Loss of heterozygosity for loci on chromosome 11 p in three clinically associated tumors

| Patient | Tissue | PTH | HBBC | | D11S12 | INS | HRAS1 |
			γG	γA			
a. Wilms's tumor							
Wilms 3	N	1.2	1.2	1.2	1.2	1.2	2.2
	T	1.2	1.1	1.1	2.2	2.2	2.2
Wilms 11	N	–	1.2	1.1	1.2	1.2	1.2
	T	–	1.1	1.1	2.2	2.2	2.2
Wilms 16	N	–	1.2	1.2	2.2	1.2	2.2
	T	1.1	1.2	1.1	2.2	2.2	2.2
b. Rhabdomyosarcoma							
Rhabd 6	N	1.2	1.2	1.1	1.2	1.2	1.2
	T	2.2	1.1	1.1	1.1	2.2	2.2
Rhabd 26	N	1.2	1.1	1.1	1.2	2.2	1.2
	T	1.2	1.1	1.1	1.2	2.2	1.1
Rhabd 31	N	1.2	1.2	1.2	1.2	1.2	1.2
	T	1.1	1.1	1.1	1.1	1.1	2.2
c. Hepatoblastoma							
Hepat 1	N	–	1.1	1.1	1.2	2.2	1.2
	T	–	1.1	1.1	2.2	2.2	1.1
Hepat 2	N	–	2.2	1.2	1.2	1.3	2.2
	T	–	2.2	1.1	2.2	1.1	2.2

–, Not determined. Alleles designated in bold type are combinations that were heterozygous in constitutional tissue.

form tumors in nude mice, although other properties of the parental cell line were unaffected. Control experiments with introduction of other chromosomes into the tumor cells failed to affect their neoplastic properties. Together, all of these data suggest the Wilms' tumor cells are homozygously defective for a locus which functions as a phenotypic suppressor of tumorigenicity. Further, the data are consistent with the model in figure 3, in which cells which suffer a homozygous loss of function of the BWS locus (or a closely linked one) can progress to this associated tumor type.

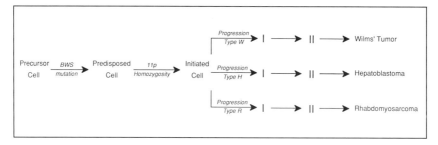

Fig. 3. The clinical association and molecular genetic similarities between Wilms' tumor, embryonal rhabdomyosarcoma and hepatoblastoma could be due to a common initiating event at the Beckwith-Wiedemann locus compounded by different progression events.

Rhabdomyosarcoma is a soft tissue, malignant tumor of skeletal muscle origin which exists in two principal subtypes which are distinguished on the basis of histological and clinical characteristics. The clinical association between Wilms' tumor, the embryonal subtype of rhabdomyosarcoma and other specific rare tumors in individuals with the Beckwith-Wiedemann syndrome and the development of more than one rare tumor in the same individual could be simply circumstantial. Alternatively, the clinical associations could reflect a common etiological event and each of the developmental anomalies, including each of the tumor types, could arise after mutation of the same locus. Such mutations could be revealed by mitotic segregation events, similar to those demonstrated for Wilms' tumor and retinoblastoma, which would serve to produce rhabdomyosarcomas which have lost constitutional heterozygosity. The experimental test of this hypothesis (table 2b) showed that embryonal rhabdomyosarcomas specifically lost constitutional heterozygosity at loci on chromosome 11p [14] and, in more detailed analyses of mitotic recombination events, to 11p15.5 – 11pter [15, 22]; the same region identified by cytogenic [11] and genetic linkage mapping [12] as containing the BWS lesion. Further, examination of allelic combinations of loci in the 11p genomic region in a smaller number of hepatoblastomas (table 2c) and adrenal cortical carcinomas (our unpublished results) showed identical losses of heterozygosity. One reasonable interpretation of this data is that the BWS lesion by itself can effect the transformation of four entirely different tissues. Alternatively, and perhaps more likely, the BWS mutation may effect the orgnismal malformations and such growth perturbation could prompt cells of the various lineages to undergo progressional alteration specific to each as schematically illustrated in figure 3. The resolution of these questions awaits the molecular isolation and analysis of the relevant genomic regions.

Conclusions

The approach described here, which relies on tumor-specific chromosomal alterations, has proven quite useful in defining the various stages of cancer development. The challenge now is to exploit the identification of these genetic changes for the prognostic, diagnostic or perhaps, therapeutic benefit of affected individuals. The rapid and continuing development of biological tools promises such utility in the foreseeable future.

References

1   Knudson AG Jr: Mutation and cancer: statistically study of retinoblastoma. Proc Natl Acad Sci USA 1971;68:820–823.
2   Klein G: The approaching era of the tumor suppressor genes. Science 1987; 238:1539–1545.
3   Nowell PC: The clonal evolution of tumor cell populations. Science 1976;194:23–28.
4   Cavenee WK, Dryja TP, Philips RA, Benedict WF, Godbout R, Gallie BL, Murphree AL, Strong LC, White RL; Expression of recessive alleles by chromosomal mechanisms in retinoblastoma. Nature 1983;305:770–784.
5   Cavenee WK, Hansen MF, Kock E, Nordenskjöld M, Maumenee I, Squire JA, Philips RA, Gallie BL: Genetic origin of mutations predisposing to retinoblastoma. Science 1985;228:501–503.
6   James CD, Carlbom E, Dumanski JP, Hansen M, Nordenskjöld M, Collins VP, Cavenee WK: Clonal genomic alterations in glioma malignancy stages. Cancer Res 1988; 48:5546–5551.
7   James CD, Carlbom E, Nordenskjöld M, Collins VP, Cavenee WK: Mitotic recombination mapping of chromosome 17 in astrocytomas. Proc Natl Acad Sci USA 1989; 86:2858–2862.
8   Vogelstein B, Fearon ER, Hamilton SR, Kern SE, Preisinger C, Leppert M, Nakamura Y, White R, Smits AMM, Bos JL: Genetic alterations during colorectal tumor development. New Engl J Med 1988;319:525–532.
9   Sotelo-Avila C, Gooch M: Neoplasms associated with the Beckwith-Wiedemann syndrome. Perspect Pediatr Pathol 1976;3:255-272.
10 Best LG, Hoekstra RE: Wiedemann-Beckwith Syndrome: autosomal-dominant inheritance in a family. Am J Med Genet 1981;9:291–299.
11 Turleau C, de Grouchy J, Chavin-Colin F, Martelli H, Voyer M, Charlas R: Trisomy 11p15 and Beckwith-Wiedemann syndrome. A reprot of two cases. Hum Genet 1984; 67:219–221.

12 Koufos A, Grundy P, Morgan K, Aleck K, Hadro T, Lampkin B, Kalbakji A, Cavenee WK: Familial Wiedemann-Beckwith syndrome and a second Wilms tumor locus both map to 11p15.5. Am J Hum Genet 1989;44:711–719.

13 Koufos A, Hansen MF, Lampkin BC, Workman ML, Copeland NG, Jenkins NA, Cavenee WK: Loss of alleles at loci on human chromosome 11 during genesis of Wilms' tumor. Nature 1984;309:170–172.

14 Koufos A, Hansen MF, Copeland NG, Jenkins NA, Lampkin BC, Cavenee WK: Loss of heterozygosity in three embryonal tumors suggests a common pathogenetic mechanism. Nature 1985;316:330–334.

15 Scrable H, Witte DP, Lampkin BC, Cavenee WK: Chromosomal localization of the human rhabdomyosarcoma locus by mitotic recombination mapping. Nature 1987; 329:645–647.

16 Francke U, Holmes LB, Atkins L, Riccardi VM: Anridia-Wilms' tumor association: Evidence for specific deletion of 11p13. Cytogenet Cell Genet 1979;24:185–192.

17 Matsunaga E: Genetics of Wilms' tumor. Hum Genet 1981;57:231–246.

18 Orkin SH, Goldman DS, Sallan SE: Development of homozygosity for chromosome 11p markers in Wilms' tumor. Nature 1984;309:712–714.

19 Reeves AP, Housiaux PJ, Gardner RJ, Chewings WE, Grindley RM, Millow LJ: Loss of a Harvey ras allele in sporadic Wilms' tumor. Nature 1984;209:174–176.

20 Fearon ER, Vogelstein B, Feinberg AP: Somatic deletion and duplication of genes on chromosome 11 in Wilms' tumor. Nature 1984;209:176–178.

21 Weissmann BE, Saxon PJ, Pasquale SR, Jones GR, Geiser AG, Stanbridge EJ: Introduction of a normal human chromosome 11 into a Wilms' tumor cell line controls its tumorigenic expression. Science 1987;236:175–180.

22 Scrable JH, Witte D, Shimada H, Wang-Wuu S, Soukup S, Koufos A, Houghton P, Lampkin B, Cavenee WK: Molecular differential pathology of rhabdomyosarcoma. Genes Chromosomes Cancer 1989;1:23–35.

W. K. Cavenee, Ludwig Institute for Cancer Research, Royal Victoria Hospital, 687 Pine Avenue West, Montréal, Québec H3A 1A1 (Canada)

Contrib Oncol, vol 39, pp 169–179 (Karger, Basel, 1990)

Oncogenes as Diagnostic Markers of Therapeutic Effectiveness in Human Myeloid Leukemias

C. R. Bartram, J. W. G. Janssen

Section of Molecular Biology, Department of Pediatrics II, University of Ulm, FRG

During the last decade, various aspects of oncogene research turned out to be of immediate clinical relevance and led to the introduction of powerful diagnostic and prognostic parameter for the classification of human malignancies. Moreover, oncogene sequences can be used as markers for monitoring therapeutic effectiveness. In the following we will briefly illustrate this development by two different modes of oncogene activation observed in hematopoietic neoplasias of the myeloid cell lineage.

Ras gene and X-inactivation analysis in AML and MDS

Somatic mutations affecting codon 12, 13 or 61 of the Ha-ras, Ki-ras or N-ras genes have been demonstrated in a variety of human malignancies with different frequencies [1]. In about 20 % of patients with acute myelocytic leukemia (AML) a mutated allele is detected, preferentially in the N-ras gene. In order to elucidate the clinical significance of this type of oncogene activation we recently analyzed 79 AML patients, including 45 children and 34 adults, all treated according to the protocols of the German multicenter AML trials for children and adults [2]. Using a dot-blot procedure based on a combination of in vitro amplification of target sequences by polymerase chain reaction and subsequent hybridization to synthetic oligonucleotide probes we identified mutated ras alleles in 21 % (17/79) of primary AMLs. Fourteen mutations occured in N-ras; one patient showed a Ha-Ras and two cases Ki-ras mutations. We neither observed a preferential involvement of codon 12, 13, or 61 nor a specific type of amino acid substitution or nucleotide transition. Interestingly, there was a strong correlation with the myelomonocytic morphology of AML cells (M4 subtype of the French-American-British classification); ten out of seventeen M4 AMLs (60 %) exhibited mutated ras alleles. However, this study did not establish a specific association of ras mutations with the karyotype and immunophenotype of AML blasts or clinical features such as patients' age, sex and clinical course. We therefore conclude that the ras gene status if merely determined at initial diagnosis is of marginal prognostic value in AML.

The clinical significance of ras mutations as clonal markers, however, became obvious by comparing consecutively leukemic cells of individual AML patients at presentation and relapse. In the majority of cases we observed an identical ras gene status. However, 9 patients (31 %) exhibited clonal variations characterized by a) acquisition of a point mutation at relapse not present initially (4 cases), b) absence of a mutated allele in recurrent disease (3 cases), or c) different ras mutations at both stages (2 cases). This heterogeneous pattern is illustrated for the N-ras 12 locus of 5 AML patients (fig. 1). It appears to be noteworthy that concurrent morphological, immunological and cytogenetic analyses revealed identical pheno- and genotypes of these leukemias at both instants.

Our data on clonal variation in AML patients may be reconceiled with previous evidence for clonal evolution in almost 30 % of acute lymphoblastic leukemias (ALL) as demonstrated by the analysis of immunoglobulin and T-cell receptor gene rearrangements [3]. The precise clinical meaning of these genomic differences remains to be established and is currently being studied in prospective German multicenter ALL and AML trials. Thus far our data indicate a decidedly poor prognosis for AML patients, who are characterized by acquisition of a mutated ras allele during the course of the disease.

A complementary approach to study clonality in AML is the use of DNA polymorphisms of X-linked genes [4]. This strategy is analogous to glucose-6-phophate dehydrogenase isoenzyme analysis, being based on X-chromosome inactivation [5]. The technique is comprised of two steps. The two copies of a X-linked gene such as hypoxanthine phosphoribosyl transferase (HPRT) or phosphoglycerate kinase (PGK) are first distinguished through a restriction fragment length polymorphism (RFLP). Active and inactive alleles of heterozygous patients can then be differentiated further by a methylation-sensitive restriction-enzyme. Endonucleases such as HpaII detect differences in cytosine methylation pattern at the 5' end of house-keeping genes that accompany X-chromosome inactivation.

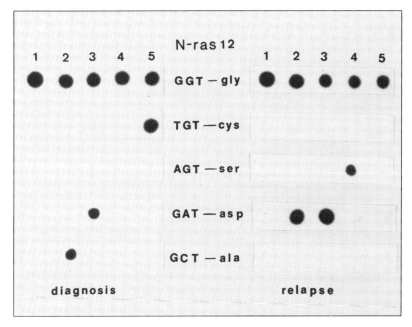

Fig. 1. Dot blot analysis of N-ras codon 12 mutations in 5 AML patients at initial diagnosis and relapse. Five nanograms of amplified DNA obtained from the patients' peripheral blood were hybridized to oligonucleotide probes representing wild-type codon 12 sequences (GGT) present in all DNAs tested an mutation-specific sequences detecting substitution of the normal amino acid glycine (GGT) by cysteine (TGT), serine (AGT), aspartic acid (GAT) or alanine (GCT). An identical ras gene status at both stages of the disease is observed in patient 1 (no mutation) and patient 3 (mutated GAT allele). Leukemic cells of patient 5 are characterized by a N-ras 12 mutation (TGT) at initial diagnosis, but not at relapse. In contrast, a point mutation (AGT) not present initially is observed in patient 4 at relapse. Leukemic cells of case 2 exhibit different N-ras 12 mutations at both stages, resulting in substitutions by alanine and aspartic acid, respectively.

In monoclonal cell populations the same X-chromosome is active in all cells and one allele will be cleaved completely following HpaII digestion. In contrast, non-clonal cell populations show equal reduction in signal intensity of both RFLP fragments upon HpaII cleavage.

We have applied this strategy to the investigation of 31 female AML patients [2]. Fifteen cases were heterozygous for PGK and/or HPRT RFLPs and therefore suitable for further clonal analysis. As expected all of the latter cases exhibited monoclonal leukemic cell populations at presentation (fig. 2). Ten of these patients could also be analysed during complete remis-

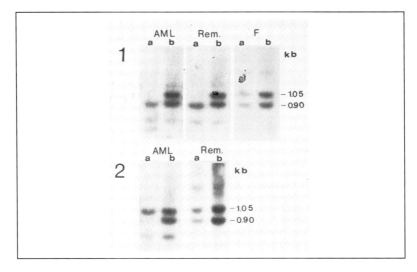

Fig. 2. Clonal composition of peripheral blood cell samples from two female AML patients at initial presentation (AML) and during complete remission (Rem.) investigated by X-chromosome inactivation analysis. A PGK RFLP characterized by 1.05 and 0.9 kb fragments in BstXI/PstI digests distinguishes the maternal from the paternal allele and methylation differences as shown by HpaII digestion distinguishes between active and inactive loci. Twenty μg of DNAs were codigested with BstXI and PstI and subsequently divided into two equal aliquots; one was not digested further (lanes b) and the other was cleaved with HpaII (lanes a). The complete loss of one allele upon HpaII digestion indicated a monoclonal cell population at initial diagnosis of both patients and during the remission phase of patient 1. A nonclonal pattern is observed in the remission sample of case 2 as well as in the fibroblast specimen (F) obtained from patient 1, used for analysis of the constitutive X-inactivation pattern of this female.

sion. A polyclonal pattern of X-inactivation indicating restoration of presumably normal hematopoiesis was observed in seven cases. However, we demonstrated persistence of a single dominant clone in bone marrow and peripheral blood specimen of 3 patients (fig. 2). Similar results have previously been reported by others [6, 7]. Interestingly, in one of our patients the absence of a mutated ras allele initially characterizing AML blasts suggests that chemotherapy destroyed the leukemic cells but failed to eradicate a population of preleukemic progenitor cells capable for differentiating into mature hematopoietic cells and exhibiting relative growth advantage over normal stem cells. We would like to emphasize that clonal remissions in AML are not necessarily associated with a rapid transition into overt leukemia; one of our respective patients is in continuous clinical remission for almost 3 years. This remission status might rather be compared with clonal hematopoiesis observed in the majority of myelodysplastic syndromes (MDS) irrespective of disease duration [8].

Primary MDS comprise a group of acquired hematopoietic disorders characterized by progressive pheripheral cytopenia reflecting defects in erythroid, myeloid and megakaryocytic differentiation. Up to 40 % of cases eventually evolve into AML. Thus far we have investigated 19 heterozygous MDS patients by X-inactivation studies. With the exception of two hypoplastic MDS variants all cases exhibited a clear-cut monoclonal hematopoiesis in peripheral blood and bone marrow samples [8]. Moreover, from four of the latter patients 5 to 7 years old blood specimen were available for X-inactivation analysis and likewise showed a monoclonal pattern. These data suggest that at least in some patients monoclonal hematopoiesis may persist for a remarkably long time without any clinical or hematological evidence for ultimate leukemic transformation.

The detection of ras gene mutations in a proportion of MDS patients supports the view that this type of oncogene activation can occur at various stages during the development of AML [1]. The presence of ras mutations in MDS would argue for an initiating step in leukemogenesis, while the acquisition of mutated ras alleles in AML relapse pinpoints to a late event. The incidence and clinical significance of ras gene mutations in MDS in still a matter of controversy [1]. In our series of 101 cases we observed ras mutations in 8 patients only; as in other studies the chronic myelomonocytic leukemia (CMML) subtype exhibited a rather high frequency (30 %) of mutation-positiv patients [9].

In any case, ras mutations may serve as informative clonal markers for monitoring therapeutic effectiveness. In a female patient with refractory anemia with excess blasts in transformation (RAEB-T) loss of a Ki-ras 12 mutation was observed in peripheral blood and bone marrow DNA after two courses of lowdose cytarabine treatment (fig. 3). Concurrent X-inactivation analysis revealed reversion to polyclonal hematopoiesis. The patient is in continuos clinical and hematological remission by intermittent administration of cytarabine. Similar results were demonstrated in three other MDS patients [10]. These cases illustrate that even at low dosage cytarabine has a cytotoxic effect. Combined ras gene and X-inactivation analysis may also shed light on the biological effects of other differentiating agents and biological response modifiers currently undergoing therapeutic trials in MDS. Cases in point are 13-cis retinoid acid and granulocyte-macrophage colony stimulating factor (GM-CSF).

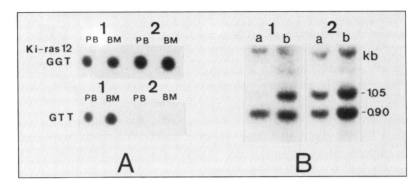

Fig. 3. Molecular genetic analysis of a female MDS patient prior to (1) and after (2) low-dose cytarabine treatment. Initially peripheral blood (PB) and bone marrow (BM) samples are characterized by a Ki-ras codon 12 mutation (A) substituting the normal amino acid glycine (GGT) by valine (GTT). Following two courses of therapy only the wild-type alleles are visible (2). Concurrent X-chromosome inactivation analyses of the patient's BM samples (B) reveal a monoclonal pattern prior to therapy (1) indicated by the complete loss of the 1.05 kb fragment upon HpaII digestion (lane a) and restoration with non-clonal normal hematopoiesis after low-dose cytarabine treatment (2).

Detection of Minimal Residual Disease in CML Patients by in vitro Amplification of Rearranged BCR-ABL Sequences

The molecular genetic hallmark of the Philadelphia (Ph) translocation in chronic myelocytic leukemia (CML) is a recombination of the BCR and ABL genes [11]. Southern blot analysis using appropriate BCR probes is increasingly applied as complementary or alternative approach to cytogenetic investigation for the diagnosis and subclassification of CML. Thus far allogenic bone marrow transplantation (BMT) seems to be the only curative therapy for patients with CML resulting in the eradication of the Ph-positive cell clone and reconstitution of hematopoiesis with normal marow from the donor. Since most relapses following BMT are thought to stem from remaining neoplastic cells escaping conditioning regimen, the detection of minimal residual disease is of major clinical importance. Unfortunately, the majority of currently available techniques including morphology, flow cytometry, cytogenetics for Southern blot analysis are limited by a detection level of 1 % clonally related cells [12]. Recently a breakthrough in the identification of residual leukemia emerged from the application of a modified polymerase chain reaction (PCR) technique [13–15]. This method is based on the fact that in CML patients exon 2 or 3 sequences of the socalled major breakpoint cluster region (Mbcr) are spliced to ABL exon II. Thus despite considerable differences at the genomic level, CML patients are characterized by similarly sized BCR-ABL transcripts. Following the generation of cDNA, respective RNA sequences can be amplified in vitro several hundred thousandfold using appropriate BCR and ABL oligomers as primers and afterwards either directly visualized on an agagrose gel or identified by oligonucleotid probes on Southern blots. This approach allows the detection of leukemia cells at frequencies of 1 : 100,000 and has been successfully used for the identification of minimal residual disease in CML patients following BMT [16–19].

Up to now our laboratory has investigated 21 cases in complete remission according to clinical, hematological, cytogenetic, and Southern blot criteria [16, 17]. Six of these patients were transplanted T-lymphocyte depleted for prophylaxis of graft-versus-host disease; in all 6 cases PCR analysis demonstrated residual leukemic cells. A significant increase in clinical relapses after T-cell depleted BMT has been reported [20]. Along this line 3 of the 6 CML patients experienced a clinical relapse 4 to 8 months after initial diagnosis of residual disease. Our data suggest that T-cell depletion of donor marrow before BMT might prevent or at least delay complete eradication of residual leukemic cells due to lack of a graft-versus-leukemia effect.

In contrast to this high-risk subgroup of transplanted CML patients all 8 long-term survivors in continuing remission for more than 5 years were free from residual leukemia. Finally, 7 patients being in complete remission for 3 to 46 months showed a heterogeneous pattern (fig. 4). Four cases were repeatedly PCR-negative, while 3 patients exhibited leukemic cells; one of the latter cases is in complete remission for 46 months. Although residual leukemic cells may indeed represent a fully malignant clone with the capacity to replace normal hematopoiesis and to cause clinical relapse, the phenomenon of transient cytogenetic relapses in continuous clinical remission of CML patients following BMT raises an important caveat [21].

Application of high-dose interferon-alpha has also been associated with hematological remissions in CML patients and in some cases has eradicated the leukemic clone as determined by cytogenetic and Southern blot analyses. However, in the majority of the latter cases PCR studies revealed residual leukemic cells [15, 22]. Thus far we were able to analyze seven CML patients in complete hematological and genetic remission following interferon therapy. In five cases PCR analysis exhibited residual leukemia. Remarkably, peripheral blood and bone marrow were free from

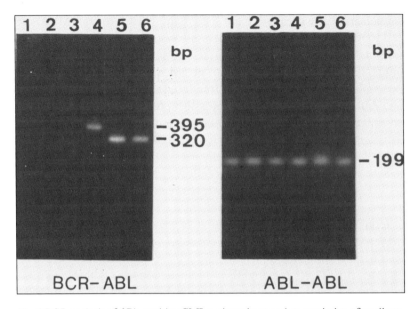

Fig. 4. PCR analysis of 6 Ph-positive CML patients in complete remission after alloge-
neic BMT. After the generation of cDNA from RNA samples of BM cells, two equal volu-
mes were amplified by use of oligomers detecting either normal ABL-ABL or rearranged
BCR-ABL fragments. All cases exhibit a positive internal ABL control fragment of 199 bp.
Residual leukemic cells characterized by fragments of 395 or 320 bp, depending on the
presence or absence of Mbcr exon 3, are visible in cases 4 to 6. Samples (100 ng) were run on
an 1.5 % agarose gel and visualized by ethidium bromide staining.

leukemic cells in two patients after 12 and 15 months of treatment, respectively [23]. Since the assay used is dependent on the presence of BCR-ABL
transcripts a negative result may be due not to elimination of the leukemia
clone but to down regulation of gene expression. The disappearance of
the rearranged BCR-ABL fragments in genomic Southern blots, however, rather suggests a cytotoxic effect of interferon on leukemic cells.
These data indicate that there might be a curative effect of interferon in
CML patients.

We would like to stress that the precise biological and clinical meaning
of leukemic cells at such small quantities has not been determined as yet.
However, PCR-directed methods for the investigation of residual neoplastic cells in a variety of different lymphomas and leukemias [24, 25] makes it
possible for the first time to assess the natural history of such clones and
ultimately to define their clinical significance.

Concluding remarks

Molecular genetic analyses of activated oncogenes have considerably broadened our knowledge of the complex pathways involved in carcinogenesis. A constantly increasing application of respective data in clinical oncology can be envisaged. This development will further improve our current diagnostic repertoire, undoubtedly establish helpful parameter for the monitoring of therapeutic interventions, and hopefully open new avenues towards more effective but less toxic therapeutic strategies. However, it should also be kept in mind that for the time being results obtained through the analysis of specific oncogenes elucidate but one facet of a given malignancy and therefore have to be carefully interpreted in the context of clinical findings and data obtained by complementary morphological, immunological or cytogenetic approaches.

Acknowledgements

We thank our co-workers A. Fröhlich, J. Lyons, M. Schmidtberger and A. Steenvoorden and gratefully acknowledge the close cooperation with many physicians, namely R. Arnold, H. v.d. Berghe, T. Büchner, J. Goldman, W. Hiddemann, W.D. Ludwig, G. Mufti, N. Niederle, H. Riehm, and J. Ritter, who referred patient material and generously shared clinical data with us. We also thank H. Heimpel, E. Kleihauer, B. Kubanek, and H. Seliger for continuous encouragement and H. Barro for editing the manuscript. Supported by grants from the Deutsche Forschungsgemeinschaft and Deutsche Krebshilfe.

References

1   Bos JL: Ras oncogenes in human cancer: a review. Cancer Res 1989;49:4682–4689.
2   Bartram CR, Ludwig WD, Hiddemann W, et al: Acute myeloid leukemia: analysis of ras gene mutation and clonality defined by polymorphic X-linked loci. Leukemia 1989;3:247–256.
3   Raghavachar A, Thiel E, Bartram CR: Analyses of phenotype and genotype in acute lymphoblastic leukemias at first presentation and in relapse. Blood 1987; 70:1079–1083.
4   Vogelstein B, Fearon ER, Hamilton SR, et al: Use of restriction fragment length polymorphism to determine the clonal origin of human tumors. Science 1985; 227:642–645.
5   Fialkow PJ: Clonal origin of human tumors. Biochem Biophys Acta 1976;458:283–321.

6 Fearon ER, Burke PJ, Schiffer CA, et al: Differentiation of leukemia cells to polymor-phonuclear leukocytes in patients with acute nonlymphoblastic leukemia. N Engl J Med 1986;315:15–24.

7 Fialkow PJ, Singer JW, Raskind W, et al: Clonal development, stem-cell differentia-tion, and clinical remissions in acute nonlymphocytic leukemia. N Engl J Med 1987; 317:468–473.

8 Janssen JWG, Buschle M, Layton M, et al: Clonal analysis of myelodyplastic syndro-mes: evidence of multipotent stem cell origin. Blood 1989;73:248–254.

9 Lyons J, Janssen JWG, Bartram CR, et al: Mutation of Ki-ras and N-ras oncogenes in myelodyplastic syndromes. Blood 1988;71:1707–1712.

10 Layton DM, Mufti GJ, Lyons J, et al: Loss of ras oncogene mutation in a myelo-dysplastic syndrome after low-dose cytarabine therapy. N Engl J Med 1988; 318:1468–1469.

11 Kurzrock R, Gutterman JU, Talpaz M: The molecular genetics of Philadelphia chromosome-positive leukemias. N Engl J Med 1988;319:990–998.

12 Hagenbeek A, Löwenberg B: Minimal Residual Disease in Acute Leukemia. Dordrecht (The Netherlands), Martinus Nijhoff, 1986.

13 Saiki RK, Gelfand DH, Stoffel S: Primer-directed enzymatic amplification of DNA with a thermostable DNA polymerase. Science 1988;239:487–491.

14 Hermans A, Selleri L, Gow J, et al: Molecular analysis of the Philadelphia translo-cation in chronic myelocytic and acute lymphoblastic leukemia. Leukemia 1988; 2:628–632.

15 Kawasaki ES, Clark SS, Coyne MY, et al: Diagnosis of chronic myeloid and acute lymphocytic leukemias by detection of leukemia-specific mRNA sequences ampli-fied in vitro. Proc Natl Acad Sci USA 1988;85:5698–5702.

16 Morgan GJ, Hughes T, Janssen JWG, et al: Polymerase chain reaction for detection of residual leukaemia. Lancet 1989;I:928–929.

17 Bartram CR, Janssen JWG, Schmidtberger M, et al: Minimal residual leukaemia in chronic myeloid leukaemia after T-cell depleted bone marrow transplantation. Lancet 1989;I:1260.

18 Lange W, Synder DS, Castro R, et al: Detection by enzymatic amplification of bcr-abl mRNA in peripheral blood and bone marrow cells of patients with chronic myelogen-ous leukemia. Blood 1989;73:1735–1741.

19 Roth MS, Autin JH; Bingham EL, et al: Detection of Philadelphia chromosome-positive cells by the polymerase chain reaction following bone marrow transplant for chronic myelogenous leukemia. Blood 1989;74:882–885.

20 Goldman JM, Gale RP, Horowitz MM, et al: Bone marrow transplantation for chronic myelogenous leukemia in chronic phase: increased risk of relapse associated with T cell depletion. Ann Intern Med 1988;108:806–814.

21 Arthur CK, Apperley JF, Guo AP, et al: Cytogenetic events after bone marrow trans-plantation for chronic myeloid leukemia in chronic phase. Blood 1988;71:1179–1186.

22 Lee MS, Le Maistre A, Kantarjian HM, et al: Detection of two alternative bcr/abl mRNA junctions and minimal residual disease in Philadelphia chromosome positive chronic myelogenous leukemia by polymerase chain reaction. Blood 1989;73:2165–2170.

23 Opalka B, Kloke O, Bartram CR, et al: Elimination by interferon-alpha of malignant clone in chronic myeloid leukemia. Lancet 1989;I:1334.

24 Lee MS, Chang KS, Cabanillas F, et al: Detection of minimal residual cells carrying the t(14;18) by DNA sequence amplification. Science 1987;237:175–179.
25 Hansen-Hagge TE, Yokota S, Bartram CR: Detection of minimal residual disease in acute lymphoblastic leukemia by in vitro amplification of rearranged T cell receptor δ chain sequences. Blood 1989;74:1762–1767.

C.R. Bartram, Section of Molecular Biology, Department of Pediatrics II, Prittwitzstrasse 43, D-7900 Ulm (FRG)

Contrib Oncol, vol 39, pp 180–192 (Karger, Basel, 1990)

Amplification of *MYCN* Specifies the Form of Therapy for Children with Neuroblastoma

M. Schwab

Institute for Experimental Pathology, German Cancer Research Center, Heidelberg, FRG

Increase of the dosage of cellular oncogenes by DNA amplification is a frequent genetic alteration of cancer cells. The presence of amplified cellular oncogenes is usually signalled by conspicuous chromosomal abnormalities, 'double minutes' (DMs) or 'homogeneously staining chromosomal regions' (HSRs). Some human cancers carry a specific amplified oncogene at high incidence. Particularly in neuroblastomas and in breast cancers the amplification of oncogenes has been found associated with aggressively growing cancers and is an indicator for poor prognosis. Neuroblastoma, a malignant tumor of the sympathetic nervous system developing in children (for a review see [3]) frequently carries amplification of the gene *MYCN*. Amplification of *MYCN* has been found to be of predictive value for identifying high risk neuroblastoma patients that require specific therapeutic regimen and is generally viewed as the first oncogene alteration that turned out to be of practical clinical significance.

Chromosomal abnormalities and oncogene amplification

Cytogenetic inspections have brought to light the frequency of DNA amplification in tumor cells and have provided a starting point to define the contribution that the increase of the dosage of cellular oncogenes by amplification has for tumorigenesis. Cytogenetic manifestations for DNA amplification have been encountered as yet exclusively in tumor cells. They don't seem to be restricted to vertebrate cells but have been found in malignant cells of insects as well [19]. Among solid human tumors, DMs and HSRs (fig. 1) can be found in virtually each type at varying incidence, and detection is usually a matter of patience. The chance to detect DMs or HSRs can

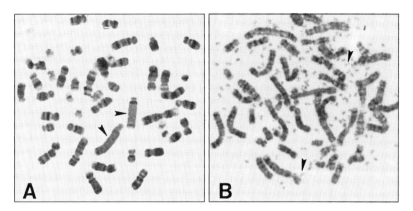

Fig. 1. Chromosomal manifestations for amplified cellular DNA in human tumor cells.
a. Metaphase with numerous DMs (arrowheads). *b.* Metaphase with two HSRs (arrowheads).

be increased when tumor cells are established in culture and when cells carrying amplification are selected for. In no instance has amplification been found as a tissue culture artefact. Detection of DMs and HSRs in direct preparations of cells of solid tumors often is difficult. This may be either due to the general difficulty for generating good karyotypes of cells of solid tumors, but could also be due to variation among members of the tumor cell population. For instance, growth of cells in peripheral regions of the tumor could be subjected to selective forces different from those in a more central environment. Failure to detect amplified DNA in a particular type of tumor by analyzing DNA with known gene probes does not exclude the presence of amplified DNA. We should be open to the possibility that the human genome contains genes involved in growth gontrol in addition to the around 50 that have been identified and designated 'cellular onco-genes'. Identifying and defining amplified DNA in tumor cells could be a strategy for isolating additional cellular genes controlling cellular growth and possibly tumorigenesis.

There are several types of human tumors in which amplification has been found at high frequency in direct tissue preparations and for which the possible role of the amplified gene has been examined in greater detail. The first setting was human neuroblastoma of which a large fraction carries a close kin of the gene *MYC* termed *MYCN* in amplified form (for a review see [30]). More recently it was discovered, that a significant number of human mammary cancers carries an amplified relative of the *EGFR* gene termed *ERB*B2 [37], which is often referred to as HER-2/*neu.*

MYCN amplification in neuroblastomas

MYCN was the first amplified oncogene that turned out to be of clinical significance due to its association with aggressively growing tumor phenotypes (for a review see [30]). *MYCN* was originally identified when human neuroblastoma cells showing DMs or HSRs were analyzed with various oncogene probes [15, 27]. These surveys quickly established that, with few exceptions, cultured neuroblastoma cell lines carry the gene *MYCN* in an amplified form. At the same time neuroblastoma tumors were also found to carry amplified *MYCN* [27]. The initial surveys suggested that *MYCN* amplification was specific for neuroblastoma. It turned out later that *MYCN* amplification can be seen in small cell lung cancer, retinoblastoma and astrocytoma although at much lower incidence. As a common feature all these tumors have neural qualities. Until now *MYCN* has been the only gene, however, found amplified in neuroblastomas.

In this context it should also be mentioned that neuroblastomas have lost genetic material from chromosome 1p at high incidence [10, 18, 42] and it has been suggested that the two genetic events of *MYCN* amplification and 1p deletion are related [10]. In a recent study molecular probes generated by microdissection and microcloning of the 1p36 region were employed to identify loss of genetic information from 1p36.1 – 2 in at least 9 out of 10 neuroblastomas [42]. Only two of these tumors had *MYCN* amplification. This result makes a relationship between amplification of *MYCN* and deletion of 1p DNA unlikely.

The oncogenic potential of enhanced expression of *MYCN* as the consequence of amplification has been addressed in various experimental systems. Enhanced expression, resulting after introduction of an *MYCN* expression vector can assist mutationally activated *HRAS* in tumorigenic conversion of primary rat embryo cells [29], converts established cells of the rat [38] and of humans [45] to tumorigenicity, and rescues primary rat embryo cells from senescence [33]. *MYCN* furthermore has been found frequently activated by provival insertion in MuLV – induced T cell lymphomas [17], and is involved in tumorigenesis in transgenic mice [9, 24]. These results clearly attest to the capacity of high *MYCN* expression to modulate the growth of cells, and it appears reasonable, therefore, to suggest that enhanced expression consequent to amplification contributes to tumorigenesis. The available evidence suggests that the nucleotide sequence of *MYCN* in neuroblastoma cells is unaltered compared to that of normal cells [12]. Consistent with this result the biological activities of *MYCN* derived from normal or from neuroblastoma cells have not been found to differ [29, 33].

Clinical significance of MYCN amplification

An important prognostic variable for patients with neuroblastoma is the clinical stage. Patients with disease stage I and II have good prognosis with 75 to 90 % 2-year disease free survival, while patients with stage III and IV have a poor prognosis with 10 to 30 % 2-year survival. Surveys of over 400 neuroblastomas revealed that a strong correlation exists between *MYCN* amplification and stage III and IV [2, 6, 20, 26]. A number of patients have been identified with stage I or II carrying amplification. In all instances these tumors which, on the basis of conventional diagnostic possibilities, were of good prognosis, progressed later and turned out to be fatal. A peculiar stage IVs characterized by frequently spontaneous regression rarely shows amplification (7 %). Three patients with *MYCN* amplification have been published [7, 8, 41]. All tumors progressed later. These observations clearly show, that *MYCN* amplification is a reliable prognostic parameter for poor prognosis in patients with low stage or IVs tumors.

A significant correlation between poor prognosis and *MYCN* amplification has also emerged when patients over 1 year of age were compared with patients under 1 year [20]. The prognosis of patients above 1 year mainly diagnosed with stage III or IV tumors, is particularly poor, and metastases occur preferably in the bone, orbita and distant lymph nodes. More than 50 % of the patients over 1 year carried amplification of *MYCN*, while amplification was rarely seen in patients below 1 year of age. Altogether, *MYCN* amplification is associated with a higher malignant phenotype of neuroblastoma.

Current therapeutical strategies for treatment of neuroblastoma depend on the prognosis for survival which is evaluated on the basis of tumor stage, on the degree at which the tumor can be removed surgifically and on the basis of genomic analyses of the tumor cells. The pilot study of the German Neuroblastoma Study Group advises treatment of patients according to protocols that are specific for each of four risk groups. Risk group A includes patients with a localized tumor that can be surgically removed to at least 90 % (prognosis is 90 – 100 % for survival of patients). Risk group B includes patients with a localized tumor that extends beyond the area of the organ of origin and usually cannot be removed completely (prognosis 65 – 80 %). Risk group C includes patients that carry a metastatic tumor, or a localized tumor that cannot be removed after four cycles of chemotherapy (prognosis 20 – 30 %). Risk group D includes only patients with a IVs tumor that frequently shows spontaneous regression (prognosis 75 – 80 %). Patients that on the basis of conventional parameters would be included in risk groups A and B are transferred to risk group C in case there is *MYCN* amplification. Patients included in risk group C receive the most intensive therapeutical treatment. It remains to be seen if the same is advisable for patients of risk group D.

The structure of amplified DNA

It is the general observation that the structure of the amplified cellular oncogene appears unaltered compared to its single copy counterpart. The few exceptions include rearrangement of *MYC* in colon carcinoma line *COLO 320* [32], of about one third of *MYCN* copies in neuroblastoma line top NMB [1], and of *EGFR* in few cases of brain tumors of glial origin [16]. These instances should be viewed as exceptions, however, and all lines of evidence suggest that amplification results usually in the increase of the level of a structurally normal product.

There are few data available about the structure and the size of the amplified DNA encompassing cellular oncogenes, and what is known comes mostly from studies of *MYCN* amplification in neuroblastomas. By using random amplified probes isolated from flow sorted chromosomes of neuroblastoma line *IMR-32* [13] it was observed that the amplified DNA encompassing *MYCN* differs when a series of neuroblastomas is analyzed [35, 36]. DNA amplified in *IMR-32* was amplified to a lower degree or not all in other neuroblastomas. The gene *MYCN* was amplified commonly in all cases carrying amplified DNA, however. A similar observation was made by Zehnbauer et al. [43], who used a set of random probes derived from neuroblastoma line *NGP*. These authors also found that the amplification units in *NGP* cells and 12 different primary neuroblastoma tumors were similar over a contiguous region of at least 140 kbp encompassing *MYCN*. In line with this the gene encoding ornithine decarboxylase, which is linked to *MYCN*, has been found co-amplified with *MYCN* in only 1 of 6 tumors [40].

The size of the amplified DNA containing *MYCN* and *MYC*-genes has been analyzed by employing a procedure originally developed by Roninson [23]. This approach involved cutting DNA with a restriction endonuclease,

size fractionation through agarose gels, alkali danaturation, partial reasso-
ciation and subsequent treatment with single strand specific nuclease S1.
Amplified sequences in tumor cells, due to their relative higher concentration, reassociate at a higher rate than their single copy counterpart in normal cells and therefore become S1 nuclease resistant when single copy
sequences are still sensitive. If the DNA is radioactively labelled, under
suitable conditions the autoradiographs of the gels will reveal a banding
pattern in cases of DNA amplification. This approach has indicated that the
size of the amplified DNA encompassing *MYCN* ranged in different tumors
from 290 to 430 kpb, that of DNA containing *MYC* units form 90 to 300 kpb
in size [14].

A direct determination of the size and the structure of the amplified
DNA in human neuroblastoma cells has been done by pulsed field gelectro-
phoresis, which is capable of fractionating DNA fragments in the size from
100 to several thousand kbp. The analysis was facilitated by the finding that
the 5'-region opf *MYCN* is a in CpG island and has recognition sequences
for several rare cutting enzymes [1]. This situation made it possible to map
the DNA encompassing *MYCN* over a distance of more than 1000 kbp. By
employing suitable *MYCN* probes derived from the 5' and 3' region of recognition sites for rare cutting restriction endonucleases within *MYCN* the
amplified DNA was found in many cases arranged in precis head-to-tail
units (fig. 2). These units varied among different neuroblastomas and
ranged from about 100 to 800 kbp in size [1]. The precise and ordered head-
to-tail arrangements is stable over long periods of time and does not change
upon establishment of tumor cells into *in vitro* culture of during passages
of tumor cells through athymic mice. Amplification involves most likely
steps of unscheduled replication of DNA encompassing *MYCN*, which

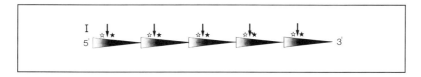

Fig. 2. Arrangement of amplified DNA in HSRs. At least the major portion of the
amplified DNA is arranged as head-to-tail tandem repeats of unit length. The illustration is
based on data generated by pulsed field gelelectrophoresis (Amler and Schwab, 1989).
Arrows point to the single recognition sequence for a rare cutting restriction endonuclease
within the amplified unit. The individual units vary between 100 and 1000 kbp in length in
different tumors. Solid and open stars indicate the position of 5' and 3' probes used for the
analyses.

maps to chromosome 2p23–24 [28], excision of the amplified DNA, integration into a distant chromosomal region, and *in situ* amplification (fig. 3) (for a detailed discussion see [34]). The amplified *MYCN* copies map in most instances to HSRs that are localized on different chromosomes in cells

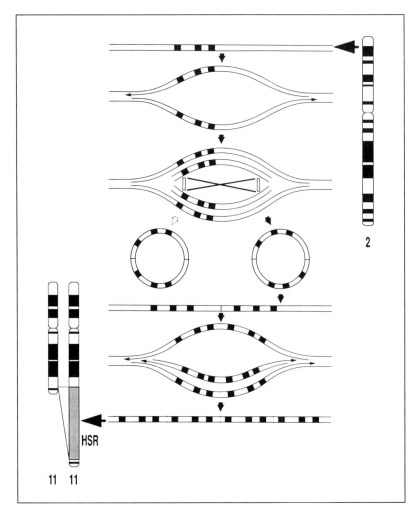

Fig. 3. Model illustrating amplification of *MYCN* in neuroblastomas. Amplification starts presumably when DNA encompassing the *MYCN* locus on chromosome 2p23–24 undergoes unscheduled replication. The extraplicated DNA is probably excised and transposes to a different chromosome (11, as the example), where tandem arrangement of amplified DNA units may result from *in situ* amplification [34].

derived from different tumors. The direct repeat structure in neuroblastomas is stable over many cellular divisions appears to be different from that of amplified DNA associated with drug resistance, where head-to-head arrangements with inverted repeats predominate and where high instability of the amplified DNA structure is observed [39]. It is not clear if these differences result from fundamental differences of the mechanisms through which DNA in drug resistant cells and in tumor cells become amplified, or if they are the consequence of exposure to cytotoxic drugs. It will be interesting to find out what the structure of the DNA encompassing other cellular oncogenes might be.

MYCN amplification in early versus late stage of tumorigenesis

Experimental carcinogenesis studies, as well as clinical evidence, suggest that the development of a malignant tumor is a gradual evolutionary process during which tumor cells progressively acquire permanent, qualitatively different characteristics [11]. Genetic instability of tumor cells has been found to be greatly enhanced over that of normal cells (reviewed in [21, 22]), and amplification of DNA may be one of the mechanisms which leads to the emergence of clonal populations with increasingly malignant properties. There is some indication that gene amplification occurs in tumorigenic cells at a higher rate than in nontumorigenic ones [25].

Amplification of cellular oncogenes is found predominantly in cells of more aggressively growing tumors, and it is tempting to imply amplification in tumor progression leading to higher malignant tumor phenotypes [31]. The reason for frequent appearance of amplified DNA in cells of higher malignant cancers is unclear. There appears to be a certain rate of spontaneous amplification in eukaryotic cells can be increased several fold by drugs, including carcinogenes, tumor promoters, and ultraviolet irradiation. These observations have led to the hypothesis that a variety of agents may induce 'misfirming' of replication, resulting in the generation of amplified DNA. It is possible that when DNA domains encompassing an oncogene locus are spontaneously amplified, the host cell acquires a selective growth advantage which is passed on to the daughter cells. Defining why and how cellular oncogenes are amplified, therefore, should result in understanding one element of tumor progression. The nature of the selective mechanisms which maintain amplification of proto-oncogenes is at present unknown. A simple but not unlikely explanation could be that the enhanced expression of the amplified proto-oncogene confers a growth advantage upon the host cells within a specific tissue architecture. Consistent with this often a specific gene is amplified in particular types of tumors, like *MYCN* in neuroblastomas, or *ERB*B2 in breast cancers. Amplification of genes could allow the host cells to escape growth control, to become mobile and invasive, or to escape immune surveillance. It is an important observation that enhanced expression of *MYCN* causes downregulation of MHC class I antigen expression in a rat neuroblastoma cell line [44]. There are alternative possibilities, though, for a contribution of amplification to tumorigenesis. A good deal of the discussion about how amplification contributes to tumorigenesis stems from studies of *MYCN* amplification in neuroblastomas. The correlation of amplification with higher malignant stages III and IV had implicated amplified *MYCN* in tumor progression. It is less than clear, however, if staging correlates with progressively and qualitatively different cellular characteristics that go along with tumor progression. Consistent with this, tumors of low or advanced stage never have revealed changes in the status of *MYCN* copy number when, for instance, relapsing tumors were compared to earlier tumors, or metastases to primary tumors. It is possible, therefore, that low stage and advanced stage tumors represent two subsets of neuroblastoma rather than successive progression stages. The two classes could derive from the same precursor cell and develop along different cellular pathways, or could even be derived from different precursor cells (fig. 4). It is still possible, though, that progression involving *MYCN* amplification in advanced stage tumors had been complete when the tumor was small. After all, progression is not dependent upon the size of the tumor but relates to qualitative changes of the tumor cells [11]. Altogether, although amplification of cellular oncogenes is clearly associated with a higher malignant phenotype of the tumor cell, the exact stage at which amplification might contribute to tumorigenesis remains to be determined and may vary between different tumor types.

Conclusions

Central issues in cancer research are 1) how genetic alterations contribute to tumorigenesis, 2) how specific genetic alterations can be turned into diagnostic tools to provide information on how to optimize existing therapeutic regimen, and 3) to open up avenues for causal therapeutic strategies. During the past decade a lot has been learned about genetic altera-

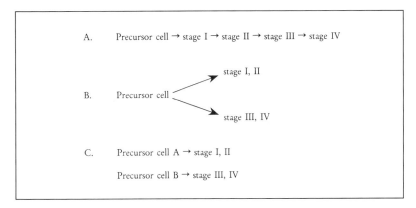

A.   Precursor cell → stage I → stage II → stage III → stage IV

B.   Precursor cell   stage I, II

                             stage III, IV

C.   Precursor cell A → stage I, II

        Precursor cell B → stage III, IV

Fig. 4. Contribution of *MYCN* amplification to tumorigenesis and staging of neuro-blastoma. Amplification is usually associated with stages III and IV. In case neuroblasto-mas of stage III and IV develop according to model A the amplification is likely to con-tribute to tumor progression, in models B and C amplification could be involved in early stages of tumorigenesis.

tions in tumor cells. The activation of the oncogenic potential of cellular genes can take different routes among which mutational alteration, translocation and amplification predominate (for a review see [4]). In particular amplification has found its way to practical clinical use due to its association with more aggresively growing types of human cancer. *MYCN* amplification in neuroblastoma has been the paradigm for the prognostic significance of oncogene alteration, and at the same time has represented the clinical debut of oncogene research. The full significance of oncogene amplification as a predictor for poor prognosis became clear with the identification of amplified *ERBB*2 in aggressively growing breast cancers [37]. The state of the art is that amplified cellular oncogenes define cance patients which have poor prognosis and require specific therapeutic regimen.

Acknowledgements

Work in the authors laboratory referred to in this article is supported by General and special Funds of the German Cancer Research Center, the Verein zur Förderung der Krebsforschung, the Dr. Mildred Scheel Stiftung, the Heidelberg-Mannheim Comprehensive Cancer Center, and the Deutsche Forschungsgemeinschaft. I am grateful to the cooperating members of the German Neuroblastoma Study Group, in particular Drs. C.R. Bartram (Ulm), F. Berthold (Köln), C. Bender-Götze (München), B. Dohrn (Krefeld),

D. Niethammer (Tübingen), H. Riehm (Hannover), J. Ritter (Münster) and J. Treuner (Stuttgart) who generously provided patient material. I thank Lukas Amler and Andreas Weith for stimulating discussions on the topic of this article, and Ingrid Ulbrich for typing the manuscript.

References

1   Amler LC, Schwab M: Amplified N-myc in human neuroblastom cells is often arranged as clustered tandem repeats of differently recombined DNA. Mol Cell Biol 1989;9:4903–4913.

2   Bartram CR, Berthold F: Amplification and expression of the N-*myc* gene in neuro-blastoma. Eur J Pediatr 1987;146:162–165.

3   Berthold F: Biology of neuroblastoma in Pochedly, Tebbi (eds): Neuroblastoma: Tumor biology and therapy. New York, Marcel Dekker, 1990.

4   Bishop JM: The molecular genetics of cancer. Science 1987;235:305–311.

5   Brodeur GM, Green AA, Hayes FA, Williams KJ, Williams DL, Tsiatis AA: Cytogenetic features of human neuroblastomas and cell lines. Cancer Res 1981;41:4678–4686.

6   Brodeur G, Seeger RC, Schwab M, Varmus HE, Bishop JM: Amplification of N-*myc* in untreated human neuroblastomas correlates with advanced disease stage. Science 1984;224:1121–1124.

7   Carlsen NLT, Christensen IJ, Schroeder H, Bro PV, Hesselberk K, Jensen KB, Nielsen OH: Prognostic value of different staging systems in neuroblastomas and completeness of tumor excision. Arch Dis Child 1986;61:832–842.

8   Cohn SL, Herst CV, Maurer HS, Rosen ST: N-*myc* amplification in an infant with stage IV-s neuroblastoma. J Clin Oncol 1987;5:1441–1444.

9   Dildrop R, Ma A, Zimmermann K, Hsu E, Tesfaye A, de Pinho R, Alt F: IgH enhancer-mediated deregulation of N-*myc* gene expression in transgenic mice: generation of lymphoid neoplasias that lack c-*myc* expression. EMBO J 1989;8:1121–1128.

10 Fong CT, Dracopoli NC, White P, Merrill PT, Griffith RC, Housman DE, Brodeur GM: Loss of heterozygosity for the short arm of chromosome 1 in human neuro-blastomas: Correlation with N-*myc* amplification. Proc Natl Acad Sci USA 1989; 86:3753–3757.

11 Foulds L: The natural history of cancer. J Chronic Dis; 8:2–37.

12 Ibson JM, Rabbits PH: Sequence of a germ-line N-*myc* gene and amplification as a mechanism of activation. Oncogene 1988;2:399–402.

13 Kanda N, Schreck R, Alt F, Bruns G, Baltimore D, Latt S: Isolation of amplified DNA sequences from IMR-32 human neuroblastoma cells: facilitation by fluorescence-activated flow sorting of metaphase chromosomes. Proc Natl Acad Sci USA 1983; 80:4069–4073.

14 Kinzler KW, Zehnbauer BA, Brodeur GM, Seeger RC, Trent J, Meltzer PS, Vogel-stein B: Amplification units containing human MYCN and MYC genes. Proc Natl Acad Sci USA 1986;83:1031–1035.

15   Kohl N, Kanda K, Schreck PR, Bruns G, Latt S, Gilbert F, Alt F: Transposition and amplification of oncogene related sequence in human neuroblastomas. Cell 1983; 35:359–367.

16   Libermann TA, Nusbaum HR, Razon N, Kris R, Lax I, Soreq H, Whittle N, Waterfield MD, Ullrich A, Schlessinger J: Amplification, enhanced expression and possible rearrangement of EGF receptor gene in primary human brain tumor of glial origin. Nature 1985;313:144–147.

17   van Lohuizen M, Breuer M, Berns A: N-*myc* is frequently activated by proviral insertion in MuLV-induced T cell lymphomas. EMBO J 1989;8:133–136.

18   Martinsson T, Weith A, Cziepluch C, Schwab M: Chromosome 1 deletions in human neuroblastomas: Generation and fine mapping of microclones form the distal 1p region. Genes Chromosomes Cancer 1989;1:159–166.

19   Mukhergee AB, Krawczum MS: Double minutes and other chromosomal aberrations in two malignant cell lines of the German cockroach *Blatella Germanica*. Cancer Genet Cytogenet 1983;10:11–16.

20   Nakagawara A, Ikeda K, Tsuda T, Higashi K: Biological characteristics of NMYC amplified neuroblastoma in patients over one year of age in Evans, D'Angio, Knudson, Seeger (eds): Advances in neuroblastoma research. New York, Alan R. Liss, 1988, pp 31–39.

21   Nowell P: The clonal evolution of tumor cell populations. Science 1976;194:23–28.

22   Nowell PC: Mcchanisms of tumor progression. Cancer Res 1986;46:2203–2207.

23   Roninson I: Detection and mapping of homologous, repeated and amplified DNA sequences by DNA renaturation in agarose gels. Nucl Acid Res 1983;11:5413–5431.

24   Rosenbaum H, Webb E, Adams JM, Cory S, Harris AW: N-*myc* transgene promotes B lymphoid proliferation, elicits lymphomas and reveals cross-regulation with c-*myc*. EMBO J 1989;8:749–755.

25   Sager R, Gadi IK, Stephens L, Grabwy CT: Gene amplification: An example of accelerated evolution in tumorigenic cells. Proc Natl Acad Sci USA 1985;82:7015–7019.

26   Seeger RC, Brodeur GM, Sather H, Dalton A, Siegel WE, Wong KY, Hammond D: Association of multiple copies of the N-*myc* oncogene with rapid progression of neuroblastomas. N Engl J Med 1985;313:1111–1116.

27   Schwab M, Alitalo K, Klempnauer KH, Varmus HE, Bishop JM, Gilbert F, Brodeur G, Goldstein M, Trent J: Amplified DNA with limited homology to *myc* cellular oncogene is shared by human neuroblastoma cell lines and a neuroblastoma tumor. Nature 1983;305:245–248.

28   Schwab M, Varmus HE, Bishop JM, Grzeschik KH, Sakaguchi A, Brodeur G, Trent J: Chromosome localization in normal human cells and neuroblastomas of a gene related to c-*myc*. Nature 1984;308:288–291.

29   Schwab M, Varmus HE, Bishop JM: The human N-*myc* gene contributes to tumorigenic conversion of mammalian cells in culture. Nature 1985;316:160–162.

30   Schwab M: Amplification of N-*myc* in human neuroblastomas. Trends Genet 1985; 1:271–275.

31   Schwab M: Amplification of proto-oncogenes and tumor progression, in Kahn, Graf (eds): Oncogenes and growth control. Heidelberg, Springer, 1986, pp 332–339.

32   Schwab M, Klempnauer KH, Alitalo K, Varmus H, Bishop JM. Rearrangement at the 5′-end of amplified c-*myc* in human COLO 320 cells is associated with abnormal transcription. Mol Cell Biol 1986;6:2752–2755.

33 Schwab M, Bishop JM: Sustained expression of the human protooncogene MYCN rescues rat embryo cells from senescence. Proc Natl Acad Sci USA 1988;85: 9585–9589.

34 Schwab M, Amler LC: Amplification of cellular oncogenes: A predictor of clinical outcome in human cancer. Genes Chromosomes Cancer 1990;1:181–193.

35 Shiloh Y, Shipley J, Bordeur GM, Bruns G, Korf B, Donlon T, Schreck RR, Seeger T, Sakai K, Latt SA: Differential amplification, assembly, and relocation of multiple DNA sequences in human neuroblastomas and neuroblastoma cell lines. Proc Natl Acad Sci USA 1985;82:3761–3765.

36 Shiloh Y, Korf B, Kohl NE, Sakai K, Brodeur GM, Harris P, Kanda N, Seeger RC, Alt FW, Latt SA: Amplification and rearrangement of DNA sequences from the chromosomal region 2p24 in human neuroblastomas. Cancer Res 1986;46:5297–5301.

37 Slamon DJ, Godolphin W, Jones LA, Holt JA, Wong SG, Keith DE, Levin WJ, Stuart SG, Udove J, Ullrich A, Press MF: Studies of the HER-2/neu proto-oncogene in human breast and ovarian cancer. Science 1989;244:707–712.

38 Small M, Hay N, Schwab M, Bishop JM: Neoplastic transformation by the human gene N-*myc*. Mol Cell Biol 1987;7:1638–1645.

39 Stark GR, Debatisse M, Giulotto E, Wahl GM: Recent progress in understanding mechanisms of mammalian DNA amplification. Cell 1989;57:901–908.

40 Tonin PN, Yeger H, Stallings RL, Srinavasan PR, Lewis WH: Amplification of N-*myc* and ornithine decarboxylase genes in human neuroblastoma and hydroxyurea-resistant hamster cell lines. Oncogene 1989;4:1117–1121.

41 Tonini GP, Verdona G, De Bernardi B, Sansone R, Massimo L, Cornaglia-Ferraris P: N-*myc* oncogene amplification in a patient with IV-s neuroblastoma. Am J Pediat Hematol Oncol 1987;9:8–10.

42 Weith A, Martinsson T, Cziepluch C, Brüderlein S, Amler LC, Berthold F, Schwab M: Neuroblastoma consensus deletion maps to chromosome 1p36.1–2. Genes Chromosomes Cancer 1989;1:159–166.

43 Zehnbauer BA, Small D, Brodeur GM, Seeger R, Vogelstein B: Characterization of NMYC amplification units in human neuroblastoma cells. Mol Cell Biol 1988; 8:522–530.

44 Bernards R, Leonardo M: Molecular events during tumor progression in neuroblastoma, in Bartram CR, Munk K, Schwab M (eds): Oncogenes and their significance in tumor diagnosis. Contr Oncol. Basel, Karger, 1990, vol 39.

45 Schweigerer L, Breit S, Wenzel A, Tsunamoto K, Ludwig R, Schwab M: Augmented MYCN expression advances the malignant phenotype of human neuroblastoma cells: Evidence for induction of autocrine growth factor activity. Cancer Res 1990; (in press).

M. Schwab, Institute for Experimental Pathology, German Cancer Research Center, D-6900 Heidelberg (FRG)

Contrib Oncol, vol 39, pp 193–198 (Karger, Basel, 1990)

Detection of Antibodies Against Early Proteins of Human Papillomavirus Type 16 in Human Sera

M. Müller[a], *I. Jochmus-Kudielka*[a], *H. Gausepohl*[b], *R. Frank*[b], *L. Gissmann*[a]

[a] Deutsches Krebsforschungszentrum, Heidelberg
[b] European Molecular Biology Laboratory, Heidelberg, FRG

The link between human papillomavirus (HPV) infections and cancer of the genital and perianal region is well established [11]. This is particularly true for malignant tumors of the uterine cervix. Within the majority of cervical cancer biopsies the genome of individual papillomavirus types such as HPV 16, 18, 31, 33, or 35, respectively can be detected. In addition also permanently growing cell lines derived from cervical cancer biopsies (e.g. HeLa) contain papillomavirus genomes. The DNA has frequently undergone deletions in different regions of the genome except within the open reading frames E6 and E7 coding for proteins of approximately 12 kd and 16 kd, respectively. In fact the E6 and E7 mRNAs and (in case of the cell lines) proteins are consistently present within the tumor cells. Moreover, in vitro experiments clearly demonstrate transforming activity of these genes in human fibroblasts and keratinocytes.

In contrast to the ample evidence for the biological activity of the papillomaviruses discussed before only little is known about the immune response of the host to an HPV infection. The reason for this lack of information is that prior to the introduction of recombinant DNA technology HPV proteins were not available as antigens in serological tests since papillomaviruses cannot be replicated in vitro and the amout of virus production in the infected epithelium is limited.

We became interested to determine the humoral antibody response against the human papillomavirus type 16 and therefore have expressed different open reading frames (ORF) fused to truncated procaryotic genes in E. coli. The construction of the respective plasmids was described elsewhere [6]. The fusion proteins were used as antigens in western blot experiments. So far the HPV 16 E4 and E7 proteins have been tested for the reactivity with antibodies present in human sera [5]. E4 was selected because this protein (or an E4-encoding mRNA) was found in HPV positive papillomas in very high quantities [1, 8] and seems to be involved in virus maturation [2]. In addition E4 is expressed in deeper layers of the infected epithelium than the late proteins L1 and L2 [10] and thus should be more accessible to the immune system. Therefore antibodies against E4 may represent a marker for virus replication. In fact, when compared to age-matched controls we were able to identify such antibodies three times more frequently (approximately 30 %) in patients presenting in an STD clinic as well as in immunosuppressed patients (age range 20–70 years) both of which are known to have an elevated risk for HPV 16 associated lesions [7]. Surprisingly, however, also in control sera taken from individuals between 11 and 20 years of age a similar number of samples was found positive [5] and even sera obtained from children between 1 and 10 years of age contained anti-E4 antibodies in approximately 30 % of the cases. Although false positive results due to cross-reactions with the E4 proteins of other papillomavirus types at present cannot be completely excluded these data seem to indicate that an infection with HPV 16 induces the formation of specific antibodies even in the absence of clinically apparent lesions and that a high proportion of young children is infected by HPV 16 presumably in most cases by asexual transmission of the virus.

The E7 protein was selected because of its transforming activity as discussed above. Antibodies against this protein were only slightly more frequently found in the group of STD patients when compared to age-matched controls. In sera from cervical cancer patients (n=120), however, there is a 15 fold increased prevalence of anti-HPV 16 E7 antibodies (21,7 % of all sera tested) compared to age- and sex-matched controls (1,4 %). In addition the antibody titers are at least 10 fold higher than in the positive samples obtained from the control group [5]. By testing prospectively collected sera it will be elucidated whether these antibodies occur earlier than the clinically apparent disease, i. e. whether they may be useful as a diagnostic marker for tumor development. Alternatively, anti-E7 antibodies may correlate with tumor growth and thus be a marker for tumor recurrence after treatment. The analysis of sera from cervical cancer patients taken before and after surgery are in progress in our laboratory. Despite the statistically highly significant difference between cases and controls the absolute number of anti-E7 positive cervical cancer sera is only 21,7 %. There are two possible explanations for this low positivity rate. First, only 30–50 % of cervical cancer biopsies contain HPV 16 and it was not possible to determine the papillomavirus type within the tumors of the cervical cancer patients from whom the sera were obtained. Therefore the prevalence of anti-E7 positive sera from HPV 16 positive cancer patients may be as high as 70 %. We are presently collecting sera and biopsies from the same patients to elucidate this particular question. An alternative (or additional) reason for the relatively small number of anti-HPV 16 E7 positive sera amongst cervical carcinoma patients could be the low sensitivity of Western blot assays which may not detect the antibodies in all cases. We therefore are attempting to replace this test by an ELISA which has the additional advantages of being less tidious and giving more precise information about the antibody titers within the individual sera.

Since human sera may contain antibodies reacting with prokaryotic proteins the bacterial fusion proteins did not seem to be useful for ELISA. Therefore we decided to identify seroreactive epitopes of the different proteins and to use the respective synthetic peptides as antigens. The two strategies accomplished comprise the expression of short randomly cloned HPV 16 DNA fragments in the single stranded DNA bacteriophage fd [9] followed by immunoscreening of the recombinants with appropriate antisera and the testing of short overlapping oligopeptides. Both methods will be described in detail (Martin Müller et al., manuscript in preparation). By either method epitopes of the HPV 16 proteins E4 and E7 but also E6 and L1 could be found.

Synthetic oligopeptides derived from the epitope KPSPWAPK-KHRRLS of HPV 16 E4 (fig. 1) and from the epitope GPAGQAEPDRAHY of HPV 16 E7 were used to screen a total number of 36 human sera by ELISA. In figure 2, examples of positive (number 3–9) and negative samples (number 1 and 2) are demonstrated. By comparison with the data obtained by Western blotting it appeared that both tests gave identical results in about two thirds of the sera. In case of E4 35 % of the sera positive by Western blotting did not react in the ELISA. On the other hand the latter test indeed seems to be slightly more sensitive when anti-E7 antibodies are measured. The number of the samples tested so far is still too small to give statistically significant results. Additional sera have to be analysed in order to evaluate the significance and potential value of both assays.

ELISA using overlapping octapeptides representing the HPV16 E4 ORF. A set of 45 peptides, two subsequent of which are overlapping by 6 aminoacids was synthesized on the tips of polyethylene rods following the method of Geysen [3, 4]. The peptides were incubated with a polyclonal

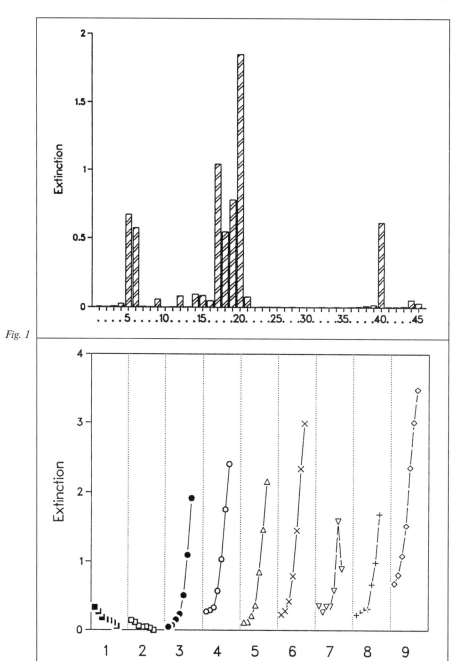

Fig. 1

Fig. 2

rabbit antiserum against the HPV 16 E7 fusion protein followed by incubation with peroxidase labeled Protein A. Staining was performed with TMB dye and extinction was measured at 490 nm. The Peptide KPSPWAPKKHRRLS, corresponding to the octapeptide 17–20 was used for testing of human sera. ELISA performed with nine different human sera (diluted 1:500). ELISA plates were coated with increasing amounts of the peptide DEIDGPAGQAEPDRAHY representing one immunogenic region of HPV 16 E7. The left point of every curve indicates the ELISA reaction for a peptide concentration of 0.625 μg/well which is elevated two-fold for every next point of the curve. A goat-anti-human-peroxidase complex was used to detect human IgG and IgM bound to the peptides. After final washing the plates were stained with TMB dye and the extinction at 490 nm was measured.

The reaction was shown to be proportional to the peptide concentration within a range of 5 to above 40 μg/well using a serum dilution of 1:500–1:1000.

Acknowledgements

We are grateful to Dr. H. zur Hausen for helpful discussions. This work was supported by the Deutsche Forschungsgemeinschaft (Gi 128/2–1).

References

1 Doorbar J, Campbell D, Grand RJA, Gallimore PH: Identification of the human papillomavirus 1a E4 gene products. EMBO J 1986;5:355–362.
2 Doorbar J, Coneron I, Gallimore PH: Sequence divergence yet conserved physical characteristics among the E4 proteins of cutaneous human papillovariuses. Virology 1989;172:51–62.
3 Geysen HM, Meloen RH, Bartelling SJ: Use of peptide synthesis to probe to viral antigens for epitopes to a resolution of a single amino acid. Proc Natl Acad Sci USA 1984;81:3998–4002.
4 Geysen HM, Barteling SJ, Meloen RH: Small peptides induce antibodies with a sequence and structural requirement for binding antigen comparable to antibodies raised against the native protein. Proc Natl Acad Sci USA 1985;82:178–182.
5 Jochmus-Kudielka I, Schneider A, Braun R, Kimmig R, Koldovsky U, Schneweis KE, Seedorf K, Gissman L: Antibodies against the human papillomavirus type 16 early proteins in sera: correlation of anti-E7 reactivitiy with cervical cancer. JNCI 1989;81:1698–1704.

6 Jochmus-Kudielka I, Gissmann L: Expression of human papillomavirus type 16 proteins in Echerichia coli and their use as antigens in serological tests, in Alitalo KK, Hutala ML, Knowles J, Vaheri A (eds): Recombinant systems in protein expression. Amsterdam, Elsevier, 1990, pp 87–93.

7 Kay S, Frable WJ, Hume DM: Cervical dysplasia and cancer developping in women on immunosuppression therapy for renal homotransplantation. Cancer 1970; 26:1048–1052.

8 Nasseri M, Hirochika R, Broker TS, Chow LT: A human papillomavirus type 11 transcript encoding an E1^E4 protein. Virology 1987;159:433–439.

9 Smith GP: Filamentous fusion phage: Novel expresion vectors that display cloned antigens on the virion surface. Science 1985;228:1315–1317.

10 Stoler MH, Wolinsky SM, Whitbeck A, Broker TR, Chow LT: Differentiation linked human papillomavirus types 6 and 11 transcription in genital condylomata revealed by in situ hybridisation with message specific RNA probes. Virol. 1989;172:331–340.

11 Zur Hausen H: Papillomaviruses as carcinomaviruses, in Klein G (ed): Advances in viral oncology. New York, Raven Press, 1989, vol 8, pp 1–26.

M. Müller, Deutsches Krebsforschungszentrum,
Im Neuenheimer Feld 280, D-6900 Heidelberg (FRG)